My new must-read recommendation—I no longer fear aging after reading this!

The only thing I learned about aging was to fear it. I heard "wait until you're my age!" or "be scared of menopause!" Outside of fear and menopause, I have learned nothing from healthcare providers and social media. Do we stop needing any insight on how to *live* after menopause?

Benfield says in the book "There are just as many ways to have a body as there are to live your life and grow older." I love this quote because it helps me continue to live my life in my aging body with my non-diet values. I know more now, because of this book, about aging and so glad a book is finally talking about it outside of just menopause! I especially love the nutrition tools to add in this book as well as the third section on body image.

This book will help me continue to challenge the diet industry. As you read this book, Benfield feels like the mentor we all need to help live an aging life on our own terms without oppressing people including ourselves in the process.

If you are looking for a book that helps you apply non-diet tools like intuitive eating and body liberation to aging—this is your book! Especially if you are trying to navigate eating disorder recovery or helping people recover, this is a must-read!

Julie Duffy Dillon, MS, D, NCC, LDN, CEDS-C, speaker, registered dietician and author of *Find Your Food Voice*.

Praise for *Unapologetic Aging*

If we are lucky, we will have the privilege of going through significant changes throughout our lives. Our thoughts, feelings, values, and, of course, our bodies are in constant flux. I profoundly appreciate Deb Benfield's empathic and insightful book for the help it will give us to navigate these many changes. Living in a toxic diet, wellness, and ageist culture, we must consistently challenge the messages we are given suggesting that we're not good enough, especially as we age. To break free from this tyranny, *Unapologetic Aging* helps us to radically accept what we cannot change while appreciating the rewards that life's changes bring us. Through Deb's wisdom as well as poignant stories from her clients, we are guided to increase our self-compassion and confidence, and to become excited about all the avenues that are yet to be explored. Finally, it brings us to the gift of body liberation.

**Elyse Resch, MS, RDN, CED-S, FAND
and co-creator of Intuitive Eating**

How's wellness culture workin' out for you? Debra Benfield's *Unapologetic Aging* offers a much-needed antidote to the toxic mix of fatphobia, ageism, and diet culture that swirls around us all. A registered dietician and nutritionist, Benfield brings decades of experience to this radical, compassionate approach to nourishing and caring for your body on your terms—no matter how thin, young, or virtuous you aren't. Drawing on eye-opening insights, thoughtful storytelling, and accessible practices, *Unapologetic Aging* will equip you to reject harmful 'norms' and embrace your evolving self.

**Ashton Applewhite, author of *This Chair Rocks:
A Manifesto Against Ageism***

Unapologetic Aging is an invitation to anyone ready to break free from the false promises of anti-aging culture and reclaim their relationship with their body. With compassion and clarity, Debra Benfield offers practical guidance toward true self-acceptance and a path to aging with confidence. She reminds us that at every stage of life, you are not diminishing—you are becoming more fully yourself.

**Tracey Gendron, MS, PhD, professor of gerontology and author of
*Ageism Unmasked: Exploring Age Bias and How to End it***

As a therapist who specializes in eating disorders and body image, I struggle to find books and resources for midlife and beyond that align with my values of living and practicing from a non-diet approach. *Unapologetic Aging* is exactly what I've been looking for! It's the antidote we need to cultivate a peaceful relationship with our bodies at this stage of life. It's a guide to learn how to care for our bodies as we age free of the narrative we're sold about our bodies being wrong and needing to be changed.

**Signe Darpinian, LMFT, CEDS, author of *A Woman's Guide to Menopause,
Body Image, and Emotional Well-being at Midlife***

This is a book we have all been waiting for. Have you been bombarded with ads for every anti-aging product and diet now that you're a person of a certain age? Instead of anti-aging (which is actually not possible), Deb Benfield brings us *Unapologetic Aging*. She shares from her decades of clinical experience a hopeful view of our relationship with our aging bodies – one where, instead of chasing endless unrealistic expectations (fueled by capitalism), we embrace our most authentic selves. What a different world it would be if we honored and cared for our bodies as we age instead of demeaning or restricting them. If you struggle to be unapologetic in your aging (and it's hard not to in this culture), you must read this book. Then, please buy one for all of your friends. We change this ageist culture with ripples of understanding and compassion. Let's change the conversations around growing older and get wiser together. This book is a brilliant invitation to embrace body liberation and joy, at any age.

Heidi Schauster, MS, RD, CEDS-C, SEP, author of *Nourish: How to Heal Your Relationship with Food, Body*, and *Self and Nurture: How to Raise Kids Who Love Food, Their Bodies, and Themselves*

Unapologetic Aging is a brilliant resource for women as we consider our relationship with food, our bodies, our unique histories, and our desired futures. I loved the stories, the practical prompts, and the compassionate and wise guidance. Incredible!

Jennifer L. Gaudiani, MD, CEDS-C, FAED, founder and medical director of the Gaudiani Clinic, author of *Sick Enough: A Guide to the Medical Complications of Eating Disorders and Malnutrition*

Two books for the price of one? *Unapologetic Aging* is just that. Benfield starts by poignantly describing how the body-shaming messages of today's anti-aging, weight loss, wellness, fitness, and beauty industries intensify racism, oppression, patriarchy, and diet culture. Relentlessly preying on women and teaching us to look at and loathe our bodies but never to live in and love them, our self- respect is stolen, and our nervous systems dysregulated. Later chapters draw from Benfield's decades of experience helping people navigate this toxic culture, demonstrating how to create a respectful and embodied partnership with our bodies.

Unapologetic Aging is a must-read for any woman who wants to understand and to revise her body story—a gift that women desperately need today. Think of all the women you know who yearn to make peace with their bodies—I have a long list of my own. My recommendation—get it for yourself and give it to all those other women too! We could change our world, and our bodies would thank us! It's never too late.

Margo Maine, PhD, FAED, CEDS, clinical psychologist, founder and former advisor of the National Eating Disorders Association and fellow of the Academy for Eating Disorders and author of *Pursuing Perfection: Eating Disorders, Body Myths, and Women at Midlife and Beyond; Treatment of Eating Disorders: Bridging the Research-practice Gap; Effective Clinical Practice in the Treatment of Eating Disorders; The Body Myth; Father Hunger; and Body Wars*

Unapologetic Aging

How to Mend and Nourish Your Relationship with Your Body

DEB BENFIELD

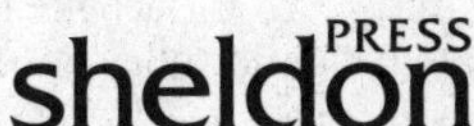

First published in Great Britain by Sheldon Press in 2025
An imprint of John Murray Press

4

Copyright © Deb Benfield 2025

The right of Deb Benfield to be identified as the Author of the Work has
been asserted by her in accordance with the Copyright, Designs and Patents
Act 1988.

This book is for information or educational purposes only and is not intended
to act as a substitute for medical advice or treatment. Any person with a
condition requiring medical attention should consult a qualified medical
practitioner or suitable therapist.

A CIP catalogue record for this title is available from the British Library
Library of Congress Control Number: 2025934249

Trade Paperback ISBN 978 1 399 81945 9
ebook ISBN 978 1 399 81946 6

Typeset by KnowledgeWorks Global Ltd.

Printed and bound in the United States of America

John Murray Press policy is to use papers that are natural, renewable and
recyclable products and made from wood grown in sustainable forests.
The logging and manufacturing processes are expected to conform to the
environmental regulations of the country of origin.

John Murray Press
Carmelite House
50 Victoria Embankment
London EC4Y 0DZ

www.sheldonpress.co.uk
John Murray Press, part of Hodder & Stoughton Limited
An Hachette UK company

The authorised representative in the EEA is Hachette Ireland, 8 Castlecourt Centre,
Dublin 15, D15 XTP3, Ireland (email: info@hbgi.ie)

*For Chloe and Bridget, may you feel free and at ease in your body,
just as you are, all of your days.*

"To lose confidence in one's body is to lose confidence in oneself."

Simone de Beauvoir

Contents

Introduction

"I started my first diet when I was 14. I'm 63 now, and I am so sick and tired of worrying about what I will eat and feeling guilty about what I just ate. Worrying about what I eat is the last thing I think about when I am going to sleep, and planning how I will 'be good' is the first thing I think about when I wake up. I don't want to spend the rest of my life this way, but I am afraid I will lose control of myself if I stop."

"I'm all in with the pro-aging and anti-ageism movements. I resonate with efforts to push back against outdated messages about getting older. At the same time, the images associated with these messages lift up the beauty and health ideal of being very thin, which makes me feel so left out. I am starting to feel like being thin, which I am not, is the only way to embrace getting older and being a part of the pro-aging movement."

"I started my first diet when I was 17. I'm 57, and I've been on and off diets my entire life. I feel so stuck, and at the same time, I don't want people to think I've let myself go."

"At 13, I joined my mother at Weight Watchers and continued to diet through high school and my 20s. I finally stopped in my thirties, when I became a parent, because I want my kids to feel comfortable in their bodies and not worry about what they eat. I'm 47 now and in perimenopause. My body is changing, and I feel frumpy, just like I remember my mother looking when she hated her body so much. I don't want to go back to dieting, but I need to get on top of these body changes."

"I started dieting in college—it seemed like everyone was doing it. What started as an honest attempt at being healthy soon controlled my life, sending me to treatment for an eating disorder. I was lucky and got the help I needed and let go of my obsession about being thin. But now that I'm in midlife, I've started following a few menopause and fitness influencers and now I monitor my protein, limit my carbs, and lift weights. Everybody compliments me on how healthy I am. Nobody knows that I have relapsed and am

> keeping my eating disorder a secret. All the affirmations I
> receive for staying thin and fit feel like pressure to stay in
> what feels like a prison cell to me."

These are a few comments from people who contacted me, looking for help pushing back against what seems like overwhelming pressure. Many struggle to describe where it's coming from or even what it is, but I know what they're talking about. It's kind of a mashup of diet culture, the wellness industry, and standard Western culture, with its inherent ageism, ableism, patriarchy, white supremacy, and fat phobia. And when I refer to all that, collectively, as "the diet and wellness mess," they don't need me to explain. They get it.

If you know what I'm talking about—if you're looking for a way to care for and feel more comfortable in your body as you age without falling into the diet/wellness mess—you're in the right place. If you're thinking about what midlife will be like, or if you're already there or older, searching not just to "fix" your body but to break free, I wrote *Unapologetic Aging* for you.

And truth be told, I also wrote this for myself. I know what it's like when your body changes—even though your behaviors haven't. I know how it feels to bend over to tie a shoe and discover a new pillow of belly resting between your knee and chest, to view wearing a swimsuit as a courageous step suddenly. And I'm well aware that my body is mostly culturally acceptable, and I live with loads of privilege—more on that later.

On the off chance I'm taking these body changes in my stride a little too easily, media of all kinds feeds me words like "menobelly," "crepey skin," and "sarcopenia," creating even more diet and fitness noise and still more body criticism. If that's not enough, there is always fear-mongering about wasting muscles, weakening bones, insulin resistance, and dementia, and—of course—the dreaded risk of falls to stoke my anxiety further. Suddenly, my friends, who know better than to engage in diet talk around me, keep bringing up carb counts, intermittent fasting, and the dangers of sugar. It's "not a diet"—they're just doing it because they want to "age well."

In other words, I, too, am targeted by the diet/wellness and anti-aging/longevity industrial marketing machines. They capitalize on fear and anxiety. As a single woman and an entrepreneur working for myself, I'm particularly vulnerable to warnings that I *need* to stay well, have a sharp mind, and be independent and able to care for myself as long as possible. (Or else? I don't even want to think about it!)

All I need to do, they say, is to double down on enforcement of food and exercise rules—on regimes and products they'd be happy to sell me. Don't I want to do all I can to protect myself from ending up sick and frail? You may be targeted for different fears—you don't want to be invisible, do you? Or perhaps you've been considered overweight or ob*se most of your life, and now you're hearing that this might be your *last chance* to get control of your body, finally (see note on terminology below).

If you're like me, you know this content may have grains of truth. And it's much more complicated than anyone wants to admit. I know it's scary to think you don't have complete control over your body's aging process. Our culture avoids talking about so much of what we experience later in life—getting old, being sick, experiencing grief, and death. This avoidance creates more anxiety, which we then react to with a sense of urgency to control our bodies by controlling our eating and movement. I've been doing this work for a long time and still fall for it sometimes. I'm watching my mother's dementia take hold. I'm working on my familial hyperlipidemia. Sometimes, I need to talk myself out of getting hooked by the diet/wellness mess. I assume you do, too.

I bring my own body story into this work. As a woman in my late 60s, I'm navigating how our culture treats aging, especially for women. I'm also a Registered Dietitian (RD) with an anti-diet/wellness culture and weight-neutral approach to caring for my clients. My take contradicts the familiar and oppressive cultural narrative.

My relationship with my body informed my decision to become a Registered Dietitian, specifically an RD specializing in treating disordered eating. In high school, I was sure I would study zoology and have a career working in our national parks. However, as an undergraduate, I wanted to learn about *everything*, and I realized that studying science left out significant parts of the human story. I shifted my focus and studied psychology and world religions. After graduation, I spent a couple of years traveling, and then worked with adolescent girls who were in foster care. During this gap, I learned more about the world's injustices, especially the injustices girls and women are more likely to experience.

After, I started graduate school studying Nutritional Science to help people feel powerful and more comfortable with themselves and their bodies. I witnessed disordered eating and mental health issues in my family and friends growing up, but I did not have the words or understanding to name what I saw at the time.

The path to becoming an RD in Western medicine is firmly rooted in the medical hierarchy, which is informed by patriarchy, white supremacy, and anti-fat bias. When I was in school, there was zero mention of bodily autonomy, neurodiversity, trauma, mental health, "social determinants of health," and eating disorders. I mention this because these aspects of my work grew to become the center of my philosophy and how I approach caring for my clients. I had to discover them outside of my education and training after witnessing the social and bodily injustices my clients experienced.

Informed by my sensibilities, curiosity, and undergrad studies, I wanted to understand my clients as whole people, not just their symptoms and diagnosed diseases. Very few RDs were like me in the beginning, which made me feel isolated, and sometimes, I doubted myself. However, my clients and the therapists who referred their clients to me appreciated my approach and called me "a unicorn," which was fine with me.

As I learned more about the harm of diet culture, I advocated for what we now call weight-neutral care for my patients. Fortunately, most medical providers deferred to me, and my patients appreciated my approach, so I provided care as a non-diet dietitian. I focused on supporting my clients in developing behaviors that supported their well-being while de-centering their weight. I am grateful to my younger self for staying true to her instincts.

In my 40-year career as a Registered Dietitian, I've held many positions while growing my private practice specializing in preventing and treating eating disorders. I've worked in public health, behavioral health, research, university health, and academia. However, my true love was always treating and preventing eating disorders.

When I turned 60, I also became a grandmother. I wanted to have the vitality and stamina to pursue the adventures I dreamed of, be engaged in my grandchildren's lives, and have energy for my work. Curious about the most up-to-date recommendations for nutrition and movement at this stage of life, I researched nutrition and exercise for those 60+. I was disappointed to find the same old diet/wellness and fitness culture mess there, along with loads of anti-fat bias, ageism, and ableism. I'm not sure what I expected (did I mention I tend to be idealistic?), but I was sad, frustrated, and more than a little angry.

So, I pivoted my career, and my Unapologetically Aging coaching business was born. With a rich understanding of diet/wellness culture pressure and how this often contributes to disordered eating, I work with clients individually and in group coaching programs, membership, workshops, and retreats. My passion is finding the sweet spot for wise and attuned nutritional choices without the focus on controlling body size and shape in midlife and beyond. I love this work and the humans who say "Yes" to it!

This book is for anyone with a midlife+ body who wants to be free of the oppressive message that aging bodies are broken and, therefore, your ongoing project. I believe that aging is living, and I invite you to consider aging with a balance of acceptance and excitement for your next chapter. Controlling your body changes as you age with the rigid restrictions of diet/wellness and anti-aging cultures can be harmful, especially during this chapter of your life. There is another way to nourish and care for your body. But if that were easy, you wouldn't need to read a book about it. What makes it so hard, though?

As we approach midlife and the onset of perimenopause, we notice changes in our bodies associated with aging. In our youth-and-thinness-obsessed culture, these changes are seen as negative or "a problem." Rather than accepting these changes as a normal part of life, we're pressured to freeze our bodies as they were in our 20s. It sounds ridiculous, I know, but that is the message you receive. "Oh, you haven't aged one bit!" is a grand compliment.

Here's a radical idea: what if you learned to care for your body exactly as it is? What if your body were not your project but your partner? What energy and brain space are freed up if you are liberated from trying to "be good" and get your body "right"?

In other words, it's possible to push back. Reading this book is a good place to start.

In Part 1, you'll get to know the story you carry about your body, along with the added layer of internalized ageism. You'll learn to untangle your body story from limiting beliefs about getting older. You'll unpack how diet/wellness and fitness cultures have lied to you, manipulated you, and fractured your relationship with your body. You'll also understand how being in midlife and older makes you especially vulnerable to this mess.

Part 2 involves repairing your relationship with your body and exploring alternative ways to nourish and move your body.

You'll drop the focus on *control* and shift into *care* through connection, compassion, and curiosity. You'll pay more attention to feeling vital and well and less to your body's size, shape, and appearance. You'll also integrate the essential element of regulating your nervous system. If that is a new term for you, that's okay. I've dedicated an entire chapter to understanding and developing practices to help you experience the benefits of developing new skills.

Part 3 covers topics that support you feeling more alive in your body. Unapologetic Aging likely includes grieving the loss of your younger body. Does your idea of growing older make room for your sexuality? Do you want to heal and repair the damage of intergenerational diet culture and body shame to protect those you love? Do you want body liberation to be a significant part of your legacy?

Each chapter includes practices that invite you to apply the principles you are learning to your life. These practices include somatic or body-based practices, breath work, and journaling prompts.

This book was written to involve your whole brain and body. It may feel awkward when you stop reading and take the body breaks offered throughout the book. At least, that is what my clients report when they are new to this process. But over time, they start to experience less looking at their bodies with judgment. They tell me about small steps or "wins," such as:

- More acceptance of their wrinkles, spots, and dimples
- Caring less about what others may be thinking about their bodies
- Beating themselves up less and less
- More confidence in setting boundaries
- Being more silly and flirtatious and just feeling less burdened about being older
- More excitement about what this chapter may bring.

You'll hear from clients who've helped me bring these ideas to life. Their stories and experiences appear throughout this book, and I've tried to include many ways to age with many kinds of bodies. Although *Unapologetic Aging* is an amalgam of nearly 40 years of experience, training, studies, and relentless curiosity, it was not created in a vacuum. It's my pleasure to introduce you to the valuable work of writers from various disciplines—and more are available in the Resources list at the back of the book.

This is a good time for me to return to the topic of my privileges due to my identity as a white, straight-sized, cis-gendered, heterosexual, able-bodied (as of this writing, as this can change at any moment) person. If straight-sized is an unfamiliar term to you, it means that I can walk into any store and buy clothing that fits my body; my healthcare providers are not going to focus on, or be biased in how they treat me due to my body size. I can fit in the seats in all situations.

Because of my identity, or how people perceive me, I do not experience what those who have more marginalized identities experience. I am fortunate that I've had the experience of learning from my clients who identify as LGBTQIA+, large-bodied, or fat** (see below), BIPOC, disabled, and gender-nonconforming. However, I do not have the experience of living with these identities or bodies that fit these descriptions. Therefore, I may miss or misinterpret information. I take responsibility for these errors now. I am continuing to evolve and am a work in progress.

Yes, this process of aging with body liberation requires effort. It can be messy work; it seldom follows a linear path. This journey can be scary, too—you're stepping into unknown territory, after all. At the same time, it is often also transformative, tapping into reserves of creativity and authenticity you may have thought were long gone. Please stay with me. It gets more manageable, and it's so worth it. *You are so worth it.*

I've had the great honor of sitting across from hundreds of people in varying stages of well-being, with all sorts of bodies carrying a range of trauma, pain, and pleasure. All experienced some level of judgment and criticism; all had tried to control their bodies in some form or fashion. All taught me more than I can say. It's my big wish that, like them, you will use your wings to fly free—truly to experience aging with body liberation and unapologetically. Let's go.

A note on terminology

*ob*se and other words that describe large bodies: I do not use words that pathologize a body unless the research I am citing requires me to use these words.

**fat: Fat activists have worked to reclaim and destigmatize the word fat. You may have done this work and feel comfortable using this as a neutral descriptor of your body. Or you may have experienced harm intended by using this word; therefore, I am using the term large-bodied throughout this book with occasional use of the word fat as a neutral descriptor.

I'm including "old" here to encourage you to reclaim "old" in your vocabulary. Whenever you're ready!

When Our Bodies Become as Linen

Cathi Rae, Ph.D. Poet and author of *Your Cleaner Hates You*

When our bodies become our favourite fabric…
says someone on my Instagram feed except mine hasn't   yet

so instead
I'm reframing this self as linen
the sort of linen
that's seen too many summers' days
too many beaches that failed
to live up to expectations   again

my fabric frayed and faded
in places so fragile now
that in some lights
it seems skin-thin
tearable and strained

and my creases won't drop out
as they once used to
despite my careful care
I run my hands across abrasions

but this linen skin
fits me better
softly wraps my body
a replay of those days
when we were people
in a picture postcard
perfect

a beach where
just for once
bucket spade and sea
were quite enough

but linen ages better
keeps pace with me
colours drifting into nothing
there is beauty to be found on a beach
of pearl grey sand and shingle.

This Flesh

Jillian Hanson

Your mind learned early to compare
and control. To perfect. To loathe.
You swallowed the con, you starved

you strove. You sucked it up to be *that*
kind of pretty tyrant, that shape of mean.
Now, you struggle just to rest and be

kind to this flesh—because enough already.
You're mostly invisible now. And who knows
how long you've got before it's *your* turn

in the ancestor museum. Still. You'd rather
recall your young mama's deer-like grace
in heels than the grim ruin of her old age.

Why is it so hard for a mind to love
a body all the way through? Not just
its slender sequined glories, but its many

fluxes. Its awkward starts, animal
endings—talons and beaks and whiskers.
Its lost bits. As it feels. As it breaks.

1
UNTANGLING

Your body is not your life's project

1

Where ageism and your body story meet

There was a time when old women and their bodies were sacred, respected sources of power and wisdom. The old woman was portrayed as a revered keeper of cultural wisdom and medicine, sitting in a position of leadership and power.

In the 21st century, these stories have vanished from our cultural lexicon in the western world and the older woman has been reduced to a one-dimensional trope. Older female bodies are no longer seen as bearers of our culture's wisdom. The body of the older woman now represents a source of fear, worry, shame, disease, and disgust and, therefore, the target of multi-billion-dollar industries. Now, as we age, our bodies are problems that we need to fix, projects that we must continually work on. It's time to change the story.

This book is written for anyone with an aging body. We are all subjected to pressures from diet/wellness and anti-aging/longevity cultures to judge and fear our aging bodies. Women experience additional pressure as we age in a culture that equates our worth with our appearance and fertility. As we age and experience the menopause transition, we sense our worth decreases; more about that later. I am highlighting this here to explain why this book is especially poignant for women, however written for every body.

We now potentially spend a third to half of our lifetimes in post-menopause, which is a staggering reality. Now is the time to stop the distraction of being at war with our bodies. My dream for you is that you spend this season of your life feeling comfortable, even confident, and empowered in your body so you can turn your attention to what makes you feel alive! The world needs our wisdom and voices now more than ever.

If you found your way to this book, you are most likely feeling all sorts of ways about your body in midlife and beyond. Many factors make us feel like our bodies are wrong, not enough, too much, and, therefore, our perpetual life projects. Adding the layer of getting older in our thin-and youth-obsessed culture is just too much. If you know what I mean, you are in the right place, and I am thrilled you are here!

Being a human approaching midlife and beyond means you are the prime target of several massive marketing machines. These machines tell you that you need to spend your time, money, and energy fixing your body. This relentless barrage from the anti-aging/longevity and diet/wellness industries does us a great deal of harm. Mass marketing makes us look at our bodies as objects to judge, fear, and fix. When we look *at* our bodies as objects, we lose the experience of living *in* our bodies. Objectifying our bodies disrupts our embodiment. We lose a healthy connection with our wild and wise bodies. In the first part of this book, we will discuss recognizing and reframing these damaging messages, in both our external and internal worlds.

Throughout this book, my voice will toggle between fiercely encouraging you to divest from oppressive anti-aging and diet/ wellness culture, on the one hand, to cultivating a softer, compassionate curiosity as you turn toward caring for your unique body. Part 1 is designed to dismantle the social narratives you likely inherited about your body, starting with your body story. This story has roots in your family, experiences, surroundings, and the cultural messages you internalized.

Your body story

You carry a story about your body that you've inherited throughout your lifetime. The experiences contributing to your story may be obvious, subtle, or completely outside your awareness. Before birth, your parents' environments and life stressors affected your body and mind. Even your birth experience impacted your nervous system and, therefore, your ability to feel safe in your body and the world.

The genetics you inherited, such as neurodiversity, and the bigger picture epigenetics, such as generational trauma, both affect how you relate to eating and your body. These circumstances, along with your environment, including your caregiver's nervous system and how you were nourished and cared for, influence your body's nervous system and neurological development. I'm painting this picture to say your ability to connect with your body and notice your appetite was underway well before you were aware of your body and eating.

Were you nourished and cared for in your childhood in a way that noticed, respected, and honored your expression of hunger and satisfaction? Did you have access to food, did your caregiver have enough time to prepare it, and did you have someone attending to your hunger? You may or may not have inherited a sense that your body could be trusted, that you could feel safe and secure in your body, and feel secure in the fact that you would be fed. Certainly, those entrusted with your care had their own stories about food and their bodies, which may have altered how you were fed and what you learned about what it means to have a body and to eat.

I've heard thousands of stories in my career from clients who carried hurtful memories for years or their entire lives. One client received SlimFast for her seventh birthday from a beloved uncle. Another client received facial reconstruction at the hands of her own surgeon father before she left for college. Yet another client received breast augmentation for her eighteenth birthday. Countless clients have stories about being bribed to meet weight loss goals as children, being weighed publicly in elementary school, and being fat-shamed in doctors' offices.

Growing up, you entered school systems and had relationships with friends, teachers, and maybe coaches or dance instructors. The people you engaged with all had relationships with their own bodies and had opinions about bodies, food, eating, and movement. Over time, you likely experienced comments from others, and, depending on how sensitive and intuitive you are, you internalized these judgments and values to some extent. You probably also received comments about your eating, your body's abilities, and your precious body. Over your lifetime, you've been building a story about your body from all of these sources and experiences.

We can't ignore the fact that we are living in a cultural body hierarchy that values the white, thin, young, neuronormative, fit, able-bodied, cis-gendered, heterosexual, Judeo-Christian, and male body above others. In her powerful book, *The Body Is Not an Apology*, Sonya Renee Taylor calls this "the default body." When you identify as other than the default body, you are pushed to the margins. Chapter 2 will tell you more about the default body and our culture's body hierarchy. For now, consider that being born with or developing an identity that does or does not fit into your culture's default body contributes to your body story, too.

You have been breathing in messages about your body from (or even before) your first breath. You are living in a body that is traveling in and out of social systems based on your race, body size, age, ability, family, marital status, social status, religion, gender identity, mental well-being, citizenship, physical well-being, financial well-being, and sexuality. This mish-mash of parts of your identity leaves subtle and clear imprints on your relationship with your body.

Collecting and carrying around these stories can feel terribly heavy. If you are ready to let go of these burdens, you are in the right place.

Embodiment breaks

I've included Embodiment Breaks for you throughout this book. Embodiment breaks are a chance to remember that you live this life in a body. Take a moment to notice where your body is making contact with a surface, perhaps your feet, seat, or back. Allow yourself to feel held and supported by the earth. If you are comfortable noticing your breath, please do so. It may help to place your hands over your heart and feel the warmth of your own touch.

Do you feel anything may have shifted in your body since you started reading this chapter? Scan your body for places that may feel like you are bracing or holding old patterns and try to release the holding and soften there. Can you soften your belly? Can you soften around your eyes? Can you drop your shoulders any amount? Wiggle your jaws and drop your tongue away from the roof of your mouth.

Please note: if this is uncomfortable for you, pass on this exercise. I know you know this, but this is just a reminder that everything here is optional. It is your choice.

Look around the room and check in with your senses. What do you see? What do you hear? What do you smell? What do you taste (we all carry a taste in our mouths)? What can you touch? If you feel stirred up or dysregulated, please care for yourself in ways that remind you that you are safe. You are here, in the present, and you are okay. You will find these embodiment practices in the Resources section. I encourage you to use them often.

Each chapter offers journaling prompts to help you become aware of long-standing and deeply held beliefs about yourself that likely no longer serve you. Please know that most of our thought and behavior patterns stem from what we learned at an early age. Some may have occurred later due to experiences or relationships that transformed our relationship with ourselves. All are rooted in a need to protect yourself.

It may feel like you are digging through layers of rock with a grapefruit spoon. Please be patient, dog ear a page, and return when you feel like you have more energy for this process. If you feel that resistance, hold it with as much compassion as you would your child self or a younger version of you. Can you see yourself, arms folded over your chest, saying, "I don't want to, and you can't make me!"? That's okay; there is protective wisdom in resistance, too. Take your time and be gentle with yourself. Your answers may come in whispers.

> Love is experienced as attention. Giving yourself your own attention is a powerful beginning to the mending offered in this book. You will be reminded of this again and again.

Start with what comes easily and return to things that feel too hard. You are not being graded or given any stars. You can't do this perfectly. You also can't mess this up. We might as well start here with the concept of good enough. Striking the middle is plenty good and often the wisest place to be. The fact that you are reading these words means there is part of you that is feeling called to mend your relationship with your body, which is the most important thing to remember. Small steps, dear reader.

Your body story is a set of beliefs about your body based on your life experiences from birth through the present. What you believe about your body is influenced by all kinds of people in your life. One of the strongest sources of these messages is your early caregivers or family of origin, who were processing their own body stories, which they inherited. Our culture, life events, experiences, and relationships also alter our body stories. Some are damaging, some are neutral, and some are healing.

Try responding to these questions as you write your body story. It may be helpful to break your responses into the periods of time that make up your life up to now: early childhood, elementary, middle, and high school, and then perhaps decades from there, such as your 20s, 30s, etc.

Here are some things to consider as you construct your body story.

- What childhood messages do you remember hearing about hunger? Food? Bodies? Exercise?
- What about your body? Do you remember any particular messages?
- Were you encouraged to trust your body and your ability to regulate your eating?
- Did you receive any particular messages that made you attribute fear or magical powers to food, eating, or exercise?
- Do you remember how your body felt at your family's dinner or kitchen table or wherever your family ate?
- Our culture values white/thin/fit, etc.—what Sonya Renee Taylor calls "the default body." How does that concept contribute to your body story?
- Did you get the message there was anything "wrong" with your body?
- What were you supposed to do about that (the project)?
- When did you feel most at peace with your body? When did you feel the most conflicted?
- What message did you hear *about* your body from people who (obviously) didn't live in it?
- What does your body story owe to diet/wellness culture?
- What is your first memory of learning that some bodies are valued more than others?

And today, what is the story you tell yourself about your body?

- How do you speak to yourself when you are getting dressed?
- What do you say to yourself when you are shopping for clothing?
- What do you say to yourself before an appointment with your healthcare provider?

- Who/What makes you feel powerful in your body?
- Who/What makes you feel comfortable in your body?
- Who/What makes you feel more connected to your body?
- Who/What brings up judgmental thoughts about your body?
- Who/What brings your body joy and pleasure?
- How do you talk to yourself about grocery shopping, cooking, ordering food, and eating?
- How do you talk to yourself about movement?
- What do you say to yourself about rest?

After making this list, consider any changes you want to make in how you spend your time, who you want to spend your time with, how you talk to yourself, and how you set boundaries. This is just a starting point.

You will be encouraged to circle back and reconsider some of these questions as you progress through this book. I recommend using a journal dedicated to your Unapologetic Aging journey. This will allow you to review previous entries and see your progress over time. It is so important to acknowledge and celebrate your victories, no matter how small! This is just the beginning. You may already sense that you no longer hold some of the beliefs about your body from earlier in your life. Our bodies change, and our beliefs evolve, so your story about your body is also in flux. You are poised at the beginning of a transformational journey.

> It is never too late, and you are never too old to mend your relationship with your body.

This book will also offer practices to help you notice more about yourself and your experiences, along with small steps to help you make changes that mend your relationship with your body and how you care for yourself. The goal is to support you as you liberate yourself from the limiting beliefs of our culture and build a partnership with your body, especially in this precious chapter of your life.

You may be starting to realize how much of your life you've been worrying about your body and how many experiences have contributed to a complex body story. You are not alone! Here's a story from one of my clients about how she learned to look at her body as a project.

Andi's body story

When she began working with me, Andi was 57 years old. Her body story began with memories from early childhood when she was about four or five years old. Her mother was getting dressed, standing in her walk-in closet before a full-length mirror. She asked Andi, "Do you think I look fat?"

In her retelling to me, Andi said, "I wasn't sure what fat really meant, but somehow, I knew the right answer to that question." As a sensitive and intuitive kid, she already understood that her mother did not want to be fat and that her mother's mood would be affected by Andi's assessment of her body. Andi knew that she would please her mother and feel loved and safe if she told her mother that she did not think she was fat.

Andi was learning several lessons:

1   Grown-ups, maybe especially women, look at their bodies to know their value in the world.
2   Grown-ups, maybe especially women, don't want their bodies to look fat.
3   Her mother would be pleased if told she did not look fat, so how you look is so important that it can make you happy or unhappy.
4   Having a fat body is bad.
5   Having a thin body is good.
6   She needs to be concerned about her own body and its fatness.
7   If she gets fat, her mother will not be pleased.

In early elementary school, Andi went to her pediatrician. Her mother was worried about her child developing diabetes (although Andi has never had diabetes). During the visit, her doctor said she needed to "stay away from sugar."

Andi learned that her body was a problem and that she needed to "control" her body by controlling her eating. She then grew up being fed differently than her brother, who "could eat whatever he wanted," while she was rarely allowed desserts or treats. Because of this restriction, Andi would sneak and hide food under her bed until she was caught. As she got older, she became much more sophisticated about hiding food from her mom.

Andi's mom was "always on a diet." Therefore, so was Andi. She joined her mom at Weight Watchers meetings and tried hard to "be good" when her mom was also "being good" on her diet. When Andi left home for college, she enjoyed the freedom to eat as she pleased. She didn't think that much about it. When she came home for Thanksgiving during her freshman year, the first words out of her mother's mouth were that she had put on a few pounds. So Andi joined Weight Watchers on her own this time.

Andi continued on and off diets through college and graduate school, where she studied to become a nurse practitioner. In grad school, she joined CrossFit and got very involved in the culture that recommended a specific diet which relied on food journaling, making macronutrient goals, and restricting food. Like most of her new CrossFit friends, she allowed herself a weekly cheat day. Her eating soon followed a cycle of rigid restriction followed by chaotic binge eating, then back to restriction. This fitness plan also required frequent weighing and measuring of her body, so she became much more obsessed with her body's size and shape.

When she started her professional life, she developed a reputation for being "healthy" and committed to her fitness regimen. She got married and had two kids, divorced and remarried, all while continuing to practice as a nurse practitioner. Through these life changes, she maintained her "fit and healthy" identity and held tightly to her exercise and diet routines.

She was early in her second marriage when Andi started working with me. She was also engaged in therapy. Her therapist recognized patterns of intense anger when her new husband would bring "forbidden foods" into their home. Andi began to see that her relationship with food, exercise, and her body was disruptive and harmful to her and her relationships.

Andi experienced a painful divorce as she was going through perimenopause. She focused even more intensely on controlling her diet and exercise as a way to cope.

Now that she was postmenopausal, she felt "stuck" in her diet and exercise patterns. The wise part of her knew that her rules for eating and exercising were not helping her but harming her. Still, she felt like she needed to hold tightly to her eating and exercise rules now because of her fears about her health and body changing as she approached 60.

Don't worry, Andi's story did not end there. We'll hear more from her in the next chapter.

At this point, I hope you can see how easy it would be to drop anchor in familiar restrictive diet patterns, even when it is clear they no longer work. You may even relate. The feeling that you are doing something wrong and have not found the right diet for you yet is understandable. Diet culture blames you and accepts no responsibility. In the next chapter, we get into exactly why that is a lie. But first, let's look at the complicated added layer of anti-aging/longevity messages.

Another layer to your body story—adding ageism and ableism?

Now that you are in midlife and beyond, there is another layer to your body story. You haven't had to deal with this stuff before, yet here you are. You must become aware of ageism and ableism to confront how this affects you. One of my clients said, "I didn't start feeling old until I gained weight. I started feeling frumpy." This perfectly illustrates the associations we make with weight gain and aging. Throughout this book, we will unpack this rather unconscious process. Confronting this may bring up more uncomfortable feelings, like fear and still more grief. Yes, this is a lot, but it will be okay, I've got your back. I wrote this book for you.

Let's clarify a few things: We all have ableist and ageist thoughts and beliefs. We have all internalized these beliefs because we live in an ageist and ableist culture. It would be impossible not to! This does not make you a bad person. These beliefs seep in without you making a choice, just like racism, sexism, anti-fat bias, homophobia, transphobia, and all the rest of our culture's values. It helps to simply notice and acknowledge these realities in our world so you can become aware of these biases when you use them against yourself.

We never really acknowledge this, but each of us will most likely experience a disability in our lifetime if we have not already. Much of your fear about aging is based on how your mind and body might change with time. That's not ageism; that's ableism because it's not really about age, it's about losing your abilities. Younger people live with disabilities, and older people live with bodies and minds that are not disabled. Discerning this is helpful so you can confront ableism and ageism and notice how they bounce off one another.

We are ageists when we assume something based on how old we think someone is. We are ableists when we assume something based on how we think someone's mind or body works. We are both when we attribute capability or incapability based on age.

As you grow older, there is an increasing chance that you have internalized these beliefs because you've been exposed to them your entire life and have likely never stopped to challenge them. We can't challenge these thoughts until we become aware of them.

One of my favorite quotes is from Todd Nelson in Tracey Gendron's wonderful book, *Ageism Unmasked: Exploring Age Bias and How to End It*. "Ageism is prejudice against our feared future self."

We can't possibly know what we will be like when we are older, so we watch what our culture tells us about getting older and apply that to our lives. Therefore, we are vulnerable to anti-aging messages.

We must challenge internalized ageism and ableism because they are not good for us. Ageism affects your physical and cognitive health and overall well-being in measurable ways and can take years off your life, seven and a half years to be exact. Dr. Becca Levy studied this by following hundreds of residents older than 50 for over 20 years. She found that the average survival was seven and a half years longer for those with a more positive attitude about aging than those with negative beliefs and fears about aging. You can find a summary of her findings in the Resources section of this book.

Overall, our culture teaches us to *look at* our bodies rather than *live in* our bodies. We then objectify our own bodies and believe our appearance equals our worth. These are commonly held beliefs you may or may not be aware of. Diet culture is insidious and teaches us that thinner bodies are more worthy. Ageism builds on this with the belief that younger bodies are more worthy.

These beliefs are learned and go unquestioned. It is common in our culture to compliment people when they look like they have lost weight as if we are on autopilot. "You look great. Have you lost weight?" The assumption is that being thinner is always cause for affirmation. The words fly out of our mouths before we even think about what we say. The same goes for looking younger. We compliment someone if their appearance is, in some ways, more youthful. "Wow, you look amazing! That haircut makes you look younger!" or "What skincare are you using? You look ten years younger!"

We've been breathing in ageist beliefs since we were young children reading stories where the "old woman" was portrayed as scary, ugly, mean, fragile, or helpless. The myths of aging are many and primarily negative. Ageism is not innate. Children learn to dislike and become frightened of older people and the idea of getting older due to these internalized negative stereotypes well before conscious awareness.

Women have a particularly challenging experience as we age. The anti-aging marketing primarily targets women. As Tracey Gendron says:

> "The vulnerability that older women face due to these layered forms of prejudice translates into being simultaneously hyper-visible and invisible. Hyper-visibility results from the exaggerated focus on appearance promoted and enabled in media by the anti-aging industry and those who have been influenced by it. It is also fostered by the rhetoric of successful

aging, which posits that aging successfully essentially translates into not aging and that objectively looking younger
provides a shield against appearance-based age shaming."

Women are also under increased pressure to remain thin and appear fit to remain relevant as they age. So, it is not surprising that when you notice changes in your body as you age, your response is likely influenced by the stories and cultural beliefs about aging. Do you hear encouraging and empowering stories about your body changing as you age? We believe white-knuckling around staying thin keeps ageism at bay a little longer in our thin-obsessed culture. This drive to pursue thinness as we age is harmful and increases the risk of relapsing in recovery from an eating disorder or developing disordered eating or an eating disorder.

We have limited data on eating disorders in midlife and beyond. When we think of eating disorders, we typically picture a thin, young, white woman, right? However, the research highlights that eating disorders occur across the lifespan and in all body sizes, races, genders, socioeconomic groups, etc. By the way, of those diagnosed with an eating disorder, only 6 percent are medically "underweight."

Perimenopause/menopause is similar to puberty as a time of increased vulnerability for the development of disordered eating thoughts and behaviors. What is going on? We live in a culture that shrouds these times with body criticism and shame. But I believe that puberty, early motherhood (if that's your choice), and menopause are times to celebrate the power of our bodies as we evolve and change. Can you imagine if we had rituals and threw parties to celebrate our bodies entering fertility and also when we became free of it?

Puberty is designed to prepare our bodies for reproduction by increasing our body fat percentage to an average of 25 percent. According to Dr. Nitu Bajekal in her book, *Finding Me in Menopause*:

"Around two years prior to the final menstrual period, the rate of fat gain was found to double, and lean mass started to decline, and this continued until two years after the final period (menopause). Women gained an average of 2.9 kg, with a 3.4 kg increase in fat mass and corresponding loss in lean muscle mass, and a 5.7 cm increase in waist circumference in the six years they were followed. The rate of waist circumference increase slowed one year after the final menstrual period, whereas fat mass continued to increase without change. Weight gain of 3–10 kg is not uncommon around menopause."

Based on my clinical and personal experience, our bodies' size and shape change in midlife. What is this change in midlife preparing us for?

Our bodies are wise, and these changes create support and refuge. These changes protect us from the risks of fractures when we fall and increase our ability to survive the next virus coming through town. Our bodies are wise and wired for protection and survival, preparing us for old age. As Margo Maine, PhD, author of *Pursuing Perfection: Eating Disorders, Body Myths, and Women at Midlife and Beyond,* said, "That new roll around your middle is not your spare tire; it is your life-preserver."

We live in a time when longevity and anti-aging messages perpetuate fear of the natural changes of our aging bodies. In a world that glorifies thinness, the seasons of life when our bodies naturally change and soften can feel confusing, even destabilizing. Living in a body that feels out of control is terrifying for some. Grasping for some power over your body during times of transition with dieting and exercise is understandable and normalized. For some, that means relapse or the development of an eating disorder.

Pressure from the diet/wellness culture dials up considerably with the additional influence of anti-aging/longevity messages. One of the wise women in my membership called this intersection "gnarly," the perfect word to describe the amped-up push to work on our bodies as we age. The added societal judgment for "giving up" and "letting ourselves go" can push us into disordered eating.

Midlife and beyond is a time when women have expansive wisdom and can tap into ripe and rich creativity. To be distracted by the societal pressure to control our waistlines is both a personal and societal loss. Diet and wellness culture has always been a brain drain. But during midlife and beyond, it is simply tragic. The supreme elevation of the young and thin body profits the diet/wellness/anti-aging and longevity industries, to our detriment. What would our potential be if we woke up to the fact that our bodies are not a problem and that we are enough just as we are?

I hope that reading this book is a sign that you are ready to question these insidious messages. The viability of these marketing machines depends on your fear of your aging body. The pressure you are feeling is very real.

Your willingness to continue working on the project of fixing your body to fit the culture's ideal better benefits these industries, not you. Midlife+ is a time when the message is loud and clear that your body is more of a project than ever before. For many, fear of aging goes hand in hand with disordered eating behaviors. But it doesn't have to. So, how have ageism and ableism impacted your body story?

Your aging body story

Before you discuss your beliefs about aging and your body story, please take a break. Check in to see how you feel in your body. Put the book aside, take a moment to make your body as comfortable as possible, and do one of the embodiment practices above or in the Resources you'll find at the end of the book.

Let's do another journaling exercise. Reflect on the moments of your life that got your attention as you noticed changes in your body as you've gotten older. Please pull out your journal, take a few minutes, and ask yourself these questions:

- How did you respond when you noticed gray and/or thinning hair?
- How did you feel when you noticed wrinkles or spots on your skin?
- Have you experienced changes in your body's function?
- What changes have you noticed about your brain and cognitive function?
- What changes have you noticed in your emotional life?
- Have you noticed changes in your sexual life?
- What are the benefits you are experiencing about being older?
- Are you concerned about what others think of you less, more, or about the same now that you are older?
- Do you feel less, more, or about the same sense of empowerment in your life now that you are older?
- Do you feel you have more resilience to life's ups and downs now that you are older?
- Do you feel like you worry more, less, or about the same now that you are older?
- Would you consider yourself wiser now that you are older?
- Any other changes you've noticed about yourself due to your age?

You are likely starting to notice some beliefs about your experience of aging that are toxic or limiting. The intersection of ageism, especially your internalized ageism (no judgment, we all have it!), and the story you have inherited about your body from diet culture creates a very real vulnerability. According to Market Watch (Dujmovic, 2024), "In 2023, the anti-aging market was valued at $71.6 billion, with some projections indicating the market could reach $120.4 billion by 2032." According to the Global Wellness Institute (2024), "the global wellness economy is projected to reach nearly $6.8 trillion in 2024, encompassing the diet and wellness industry across various sectors like nutrition, fitness, personal care, and mental health." These numbers are staggering and hard to grasp, reflective of the power the marketing strategies you are exposed to on the daily. Please read this paragraph again and let this sink in.

You are sitting in the crosshairs of this massive marketing machine. For these corporations and capitalist interests, the more you feel that your body is not enough, too much, or just not okay, the better consumer of these products you are. Understanding this phenomenon will help you understand why you feel so much pressure to "fix" your body. Let's challenge some of these limiting beliefs, starting with the stories we have about aging.

Limiting beliefs about aging

Let's review the most commonly believed myths about aging and then offer a reality check.

Older people are stuck in their ways

Old dogs can learn new tricks. As we age, we continue to be able to learn new things, create new memories, grow, and improve in many ways. Yes, aging does often come with cognitive changes, but guess what? Many of the cognitive changes we experience as we age are positive! For example, we have the capacity for deeper knowledge and wisdom drawn from our life experiences. Studies show that the brain maintains the ability to change and adapt so that we can manage new challenges and tasks as we grow older. Discovering new experiences and trying new skills may improve cognitive abilities. Seeking new social connections and engaging in social activities can keep your brain active and boost your cognitive health.

Getting older causes depression

In fact, studies show that older adults are less likely to experience depression than young adults. A phenomenon called the U-shaped curve of happiness shows we are happiest when we are on both ends of our lives, when we are young and old. However, more recent research addresses the complications of economics and privilege. Like most things in our world, health and happiness vary based on the social determinants of health, much more than your age.

Staying independent in old age is so important

In our culture, we've learned to value independence. The "strong, independent woman" and "rugged individualism" are not doing us any favors. In reality, learning to be interdependent may be more beneficial. As defined by two or more people relying on each other and providing help and support, it is a wise arrangement as we age. Being able to ask for help and to be part of a collective is far healthier than being independent. Valuing independence rather than being part of a community is associated with a colonized culture and it's not doing us any favors.

Getting older means you are no longer sexual

Yes, menopause and aging change our sex organs, but these changes do not have to affect your sexuality. Sexuality is the way we experience and express ourselves sexually. It involves feelings, desires, actions, and identity and can include many types of physical touch or stimulation. Intimacy is a feeling of closeness and connectedness in a relationship that can occur with or without a physical component.

The changes we experience as we age may offer an opportunity to explore our sexual identity and preferences. Transitions can serve as opportunities for experimentation and discovery. There is no right way to be a sexual person! Some may value both a sexual and intimate relationship, some are content with one without the other, and still others may choose a life without these experiences. All choices are valid. See Chapter 9 for a full exploration of this topic, especially related to your relationship with your body.

Getting older means being less physically active

No matter your age, anyone with most health conditions can participate in some type of physical activity if they are interested. Being physically active may prevent and help manage some chronic mental and physical conditions. Yoga, tai chi, and similar mind-body movement practices can improve balance and overall well-being. Chapter 3 explores how your relationship with movement may be complicated by diet/wellness and anti-aging/longevity culture. Chapter 6 discusses how movement can play a significant role in healing your relationship with your body as you age.

Loneliness is part of being older

Yes, growing older is indeed accompanied by losses as friends and loved ones become ill and die. Children grow up and leave home. With changes in jobs and projects, you may lose contact with co-workers and colleagues. We experience many changes and potential losses as we age; there is no denying that. However, loneliness is a problem across the lifespan. Getting older does not necessarily mean isolation. Loneliness does not have to be a part of aging, as growing older can have many emotional benefits, such as long-lasting relationships and a rich lifetime of memories to share with those you connect with. You may also have more time for relationships and community involvement in this chapter of your life.

It is important to distinguish between being alone and loneliness. Loneliness relates more to the quality and authenticity of our connections. This may be another part of your life that would benefit from your attention and curiosity. Would you benefit from more effort in connecting with others? No pressure, just a curiosity.

As you get older, you develop dementia

Dementia is not a normal part of aging. Although the risk of dementia grows as people get older, it is not inevitable, and many people live into their 90s and beyond without the significant declines in thinking and behavior that characterize dementia. Occasionally, forgetting an appointment or losing your keys are typical signs of mild forgetfulness, common in normal aging. Nevertheless, you should consult your healthcare provider if you have serious concerns about your memory and thinking or notice changes in your behavior and personality. These problems can have various causes, some of which are treatable or reversible. Finding the cause is important for determining the best next steps.

Let's be clear: your aging body is *not* the problem. Ageism, especially internalized ageism and ableism, is a very real problem. If ageism and ableism are new topics for you, educating yourself beyond this book will help you become more aware of how these societal stories affect you. I've included resources for you in the back of this book. In the remaining chapters of Part 1, we'll discuss how diet/wellness and fitness culture, along with anti-aging and longevity messages, are harmful. Part 2 will focus on your mending, and Part 3 will focus on your thriving. One of my personal mantras is "No mud, no lotus." You have to get into the muddy mess of it all to bloom. So here goes!

2

Food and eating rules—a fractured body connection

Maybe you've been trying to follow an eating plan of one kind or another for what seems like forever, and you are tired of it. The amplified noise about controlling your body and your diet in midlife and menopause is pushing you to exhaustion with this rhetoric.

Maybe you struggled with an eating disorder earlier in your life, and you worked hard to heal and put this fight in your rearview mirror. As your body has changed in midlife, you feel more pulled into the diet/fitness culture messages.

Maybe you've received some concerning health news and feel frightened and anxious. Suddenly controlling your diet and exercise seems like a great idea.

Maybe you're watching a loved one struggle with a disease, and you begin to follow influencers on social media who focus on diets for longevity. Now, you are thinking about completely overhauling your food choices.

Maybe you're starting to feel invisible in the world or irrelevant in your workplace or relationships. You want to feel like you belong. Suddenly, you want to lose weight because that might help you feel seen and interesting again.

Maybe your identity as a person who is "fit" and "healthy" feels like it is slipping away as you age. You need to be more extreme with your exercise and eating plan to be part of the group.

If any of these "maybes" fit you, keep reading.

Vulnerability to diet/wellness culture

Why is being in midlife and beyond creating greater vulnerability to diet/wellness culture? You are at a crossroads, a time of significant transition, which is at least uneasy and potentially terrifying. The midlife transition is also a time of emergence into your next chapter, which is potentially thrilling! Still, times of transformation are destabilizing. So you may feel pulled toward the promises of stability and the familiarity of diet/wellness culture. The changes you are experiencing seem to be coming from all sides:

- Your body is changing shape, composition, and size even though your habits may be the same.
- Wanting to control your body makes sense when your life is full of changes and losses.
- Your friends and family are struggling with their health and this floods you with health anxieties.
- Midlife weight gain may bring weight stigma or body shaming from your healthcare provider (and that's not okay!).
- Your friends and family are making body-shaming comments about others or you receive them yourself.
- Your health behaviors may be a valued part of your identity and community. The normal changes of your aging body may threaten this part of your identity, making you feel you "should" be more focused on your eating and exercise.
- You fear the judgment of others and the dreaded statement, "They've let themselves go."
- You may feel you are being ignored or passed over in your workplace.
- You may feel less sexual or perceived as less sexually alive.
- You may feel invisible in your relationships or the world at large.

Isn't it strange that feeling marginalized makes you want to focus on your eating and fitness? Understanding our culture's way of elevating and legitimizing some bodies more than others helps you understand more about what you are sensing on a less conscious level. It's not just you. We live in a body hierarchy.

Body hierarchy

We live in a culture that values certain bodies and pushes others to the margins. You receive messages from all sides that some bodies are good and others are bad, from:

- Providers of care
- Friends and family
- Media
- Fashion industry
- Fitness industry
- Diet/wellness industry
- Anti-aging/longevity industry.

Most insidiously, this message also comes from inside your own head; from years and years of absorbing it from others.

Our body hierarchy is a system that ranks bodies on a ladder of worthiness based on body characteristics. At the top of this hierarchy, you will find what Sonya Renee Taylor calls "the default body." Those with the default body belong and have power automatically, without earning their place, solely based on body characteristics and appearance. The more identities you carry outside of this default, the more you are pushed to the margins or seen as "other".

The default body is:

- White
- Young
- Thin
- Able-bodied

- Male
- Fit
- Heterosexual
- Neuronormative
- Cis-gendered
- "Healthy."

How much you embody this "default body" has no doubt changed in your lifetime. You may have lost weight and suddenly felt seen and more valued. You may have masked symptoms of ADHD, anxiety, or depression to survive the holidays with your family. You may have experimented with cosmetic procedures or dying your hair or makeup to look younger and gotten a job offer.

I've done small things like having my nails done or dressing a certain way, and I noticed that I was treated differently, as if I had more value. This is based on how you rank on the ladder of the body hierarchy.

As you age or become less able-bodied, you are pushed further to the margins. Wherever you are on this body hierarchy, aging will likely take you down a rung. You may feel less relevant, invisible, and no longer valued at work, in relationships, and in your community.

You instinctively know that thinness, fitness, and appearing more youthful will make you more accepted. Another way of thinking about it is that you may "pass" as appearing to have the default body. This subtle experience may or may not be in your conscious awareness. But as you get older, you'll probably want to be thinner, fitter, and appear more youthful. And several industries are counting on you feeling that way!

As you become more aware of this phenomenon, you will be a more conscious consumer of the programs and products that play on your vulnerability to the body hierarchy. Let me be clear: I am *not* saying that you are a vulnerable person. This body hierarchy makes you vulnerable to the marketing machines.

The tricky part is when you push yourself to the margins and value other bodies more than your own. It's okay; we've all inherited this mess. The good news is that you are starting to untangle yourself from it. As you see our culture's body hierarchy, you also see diet/wellness culture for what it is.

But first, what the hell is diet/wellness culture?

Everything everywhere all at once—diet/wellness culture

Many have written about the harmful effects of dieting, so I am not going into great detail here. Yes, actual research and data show that dieting is harmful. (Check out the Resources section for recommended podcasts, books, articles, and more—if this is new to you, please go there now and unlearn the diet and wellness lies you believed before reading further.)

We have data that supports the following statements:

1 Diets don't work.
2 Weight cycling is harmful.
3 Weight stigma is harmful.
4 Dieting increases the risk of developing disordered eating.

Still, despite the overwhelming scientific evidence, the messages promoting diet/wellness culture continue. We are bombarded by diet/wellness culture messages in subtle and loud, manipulative, gaslighting, and obnoxious ways.

Social media, ever-present advertising campaigns, and comments from strangers, friends, family, and even your care providers are full of diet/wellness dogma. You've been breathing in these messages your entire life. If you think about it, this is nothing new. It's been suggested that changing/shrinking/perfecting/youth-ifying your body should be your top priority, probably as far back as you can remember.

While writing your body story, you may recall family members who enforced food rules, didn't allow you to wear certain clothes or colors, or highly valued "clean" eating. As a child, especially if you were sensitive and intuitive, you took in these comments and applied them to your own body. For example, if your family highly valued exercise, you probably felt that you "should" join to fit in, to be worthy of the love and care of your caregivers and siblings. Or you may have heard body shaming comments made by family members and looked at your own body with the same criticism.

Your body story may have also included comments from teachers, coaches, instructors, and even other kids in school about good or bad food and the right and wrong way to eat, exercise, and have a body. All of that sinks in, especially in childhood. Our brains are Velcro for negativity; it has a longer-lasting impact and more powerful influence on our brains than positive feedback, called the negativity bias. This reaction is to protect us from potential threats. You may not realize how much you have absorbed until you slow down and listen to your inner dialogue. It's essential to notice your beliefs about food, exercise, and your body in order to shift and change harmful and limiting beliefs.

From these experiences, a part of you learned that you were safe if you earned your place or belonged in your community. And that part of you still wants to protect you from being an outsider. Of course, that is not true, but it feels true. That's one of the reasons this is hard, courageous work.

You've likely internalized the general belief that you're supposed to continually work on your eating, exercise, and body to fix it, to improve and better yourself! At the same time, your body is not supposed to change, ever! Definitely don't get older. This is confusing and maddening, complete mind-fuckery.

But look, bodies change. That's what they do. Our bodies change for many reasons. There are times when your body changes due to your life cycle, stressors, experiences and circumstances, injuries, illnesses, medication, surgeries, and changes in significant relationships. Remember when you lost or gained weight when you fell in love, went away to college, lost someone you loved, started a new job, or moved? And there are as many ways of handling those changes as there are humans.

Especially during times of transition, your body is more likely to change. These experiences affect each of us differently.

And then there is midlife.

What I've always done doesn't "work" anymore—bodies in midlife

Perimenopause, menopause, and growing older in general change your body's size, shape, and function. Accepting and normalizing this fact is an empowering and protective way of navigating midlife.

However, it is hard to do. Our culture encourages you to respond to midlife by pushing your body harder and restricting your diet even more. The desperate refrain I hear is, "What I've always done isn't 'working' anymore."

This begs the questions, "How long have you been striving to control your body? How long have you been suppressing your weight? How long have you seen your body as a project you must work on?"

Midlife changes are usually unwelcome and cause distress—which you might handle by trying to exert more control over your body and developing (or return to) disordered eating habits. Your body changes in midlife in ways that can feel out of control, like in puberty. In puberty, the female body "increases in body fat from 11 lbs to 25 lbs, a 120% increase, compared with a 44% increase in lean body weight. This leads to a change in the ratio of lean mass to body fat from 5:1 to 3:1." This change is normal and natural and supports reproductive health. Apart from the numbers, you may also remember receiving more attention for your body, feeling self-conscious or body shame, and being very confused. This is where you may have started controlling your eating and exercise and developed disordered eating.

If you struggled with disordered eating before, perimenopause and menopause can trigger these old patterns. This may be happening below your conscious awareness, or maybe you are very aware of your discomfort with your body changing and seeking your next diet and exercise plan to "get on top of things." Either way, you may feel a strong urge to take action to make your body stop shifting as you age.

Notes from an expert

Karen Samuels, Ph.D. is a licensed Clinical Psychologist, practicing for over 35 years, specializing in midlife and beyond, and other forgotten and invisibilized populations, and co-founder of the non-profit organization COPE (Community Outreach for the Prevention of Eating Disorders):

"Diet culture, beauty culture, and the commercial industry is focusing on menopause and trying to monetize it and capitalize on it. Capitalism at its finest. They are capitalizing on a normal health transition. There is just an explosion of false information.

Now, we've gotten in the crosshairs of the use of GLP-1s. The message is that you don't have to have an aging body. You can inject yourself and combat the normal process of bodies changing across the lifespan rather than understanding with compassion that our bodies are built for survival.

Our bodies are elegant organisms that are meant to change across the lifespan. If your body changes, if you gain weight, if you get wrinkles, if your hair grays, all these bad things are going to happen to you. Which is absolutely counter to the data. People live longer with some extra body weight.

The body changes that occur at menopause and beyond are actually part of the system of why women historically live longer. There's some research. Deborah J. Clegg, Ph.D., MBA, researcher at Texas Tech University, talks about the extra body fat in the midsection postmenopause as a "3rd ovary". That extra adipose tissue has enormous generativity components that are neurobiologically driven, and that extra weight actually is a 3rd ovary kicking in after menopause. When our ovaries stop, the extra body fat kicks in. Nobody wants to hear your body changing at midlife and having a rounder midsection, and the weight redistribution is actually part of why we live longer. Because there's nothing to sell.

We can't capitalize on selling body acceptance and helping people learn how to live more comfortably in an aging body. That's not a sexy sell."

Body break

You've been reading some jarring information about your culture and your body. Take a moment to check in with yourself.

Put this book down, stretch, or look at the sky. Take a moment to rest or have a snack, a cup of tea, or a glass of water.

As you reconnect with your body, are you noticing any places in your body that feel like old patterns of holding or bracing? Can you soften? Can you let go of anything? You will find practices that help you connect with your body in the Resources section of this book.

The harm of dieting—a fractured body connection

You are unique, and your life path makes you more unique. Your genetics, habits, diet, exercise history, physical and mental well-being, illnesses and injuries, stressors, and traumas from your past and present all converge to make you who you are in this moment. When you consider recommendations about how you should and shouldn't nourish and care for yourself remember: **you are your own best authority**.

By knowing that *you are the expert of you*, now the challenge is to connect to your body so that you can hear the information your body is sending. Don't be surprised if you don't hear those messages right away. Your body's data may not be as accessible to you as you would like.

In childhood, your family influenced your relationships with your body, for better and for worse. We now know that kids who grow up with parents who listen and are responsive to their hunger, satiety, and preferences exhibit greater body confidence and eating competence. If this wasn't your experience, your caregivers encouraged you to ignore your body's cues. They told you to eat this, not that, or eat this so you can eat that. More specifically, maybe the rule was to eat your vegetables or clean your plate to get dessert. Or maybe you were not allowed seconds of the starches at mealtime. There could have been different food rules for siblings at your dinner table growing up. Well-intended caretakers have intruded into your personal choices about eating, which interrupted your connection with your body. All of this confused the easy relationship with your body you likely had at birth. You may have experienced food insecurity at some point in your life which also required you to ignore or override your hunger.

The family table may also be the first exposure to diet culture. You don't have to be "put on a diet" as a kid to pick up diet culture messages. If your caregivers followed their own food rules, commented about feeling guilty about eating certain foods, criticized their body or others' bodies, skipped meals, "worked off" eating certain foods, and obeyed actual diet "rules," they contributed to your diet culture beliefs.

If you've lived for very long, you've been exposed to the flip-flop of diet culture dogma. In the 80s, fats were considered the problem, and carbohydrates were lifted up as superior. Current diet culture demonizes carbohydrates, and some diets encourage high-fat levels. Avocados were forbidden, and now they are a superfood. It goes on and on.

Diet culture's rules are ridiculous but omnipresent. It helps to step back and see how ridiculous the whole diet/wellness mess can be. Here is a list of diet culture food rules that have made rounds on social media:

- Eat five small meals and run.
- Don't snack; only eat breakfast and dinner and walk 10,000 steps.
- Eat a lot of protein and lift.
- Don't eat too much protein; it's bad for your kidneys.
- Don't do any cardio; it's bad for your joints.
- Don't eat too much protein, sleep a lot.
- Don't be too sedentary.
- Don't be too active; it's bad for your blood pressure.
- Replace all your lost salt; but don't eat too much sodium.
- Fruit is good for you.
- Fruit is bad for you because it's only sugar.
- Fish is super good for you.
- Fish is full of mercury, which will be killing you.
- Never starve yourself or fast.
- Intermittent or intuitive fasting benefits heart health and reduces inflammation.
- Vegan is the healthiest lifestyle.
- Keto is the healthiest lifestyle.
- Paleo is the healthiest lifestyle.
- It's easy, just eat vegetables, except potatoes and corn.
- Drink lots of water, but it only counts if you add electrolytes, but don't overhydrate yourself.
- It's simple! Anybody can do it!

Diet culture messages set up deprivation and cravings by establishing dichotomies of "good" and "bad" foods. Sometimes, influencers and diet-peddlers have clearly stated lists of forbidden foods. The experience of restriction and food rules is so much a part of your daily life that diet culture phrases are sprinkled into your conversations. How often do you hear or think these words and phrases that are rooted in diet culture:

- Cheat days
- Clean eating
- Healthy/whole or super food
- Junk/processed/ultra-processed food
- Sinful/decadent/indulgent
- Toxin/cleanse
- Being good/being bad
- "I've earned this"
- Damage control/atone/do penance with exercise
- Double down on restriction
- Craving.

When you follow dieting rules, you ignore your hunger cues resulting from your caloric deficit. When you successfully override your hunger and cravings, you feel like you are doing well and "on top of things." At first, this experience provides a dopamine rush and gives you a feeling of being in control. But then, over time, "pushing through" your hunger with chronic dieting and disordered eating fractures your relationship with your body. The diet/binge cycle is a normal and protective response to dieting. But it really messes with your mind-body connection.

Your body is wired to prioritize survival, to protect you from the threat of starvation with the feeling of hunger. It is normal for your body to send you intense and uncomfortable hunger sensations and obsessive thoughts about food. It is normal for you to eat past fullness when you become overly hungry. However, when this happens you can feel out of control and trigger stories like, *I cannot be trusted around this food, I have no willpower*. You feel that you cannot trust your body when, in fact, your body cannot trust you to nourish yourself. Diet culture reinforces this fracture in your relationship with your body and the whole diet/binge cycle is born. This is not your fault!

Your body experiences restriction as a threat, and your brain experiences deprivation as torture (not allowing pleasure). A healthy body and brain will push back and tell you to eat the foods you enjoy until your body is reassured that the threat has passed and you are safe. What a beautiful design for survival!

The problem is that diet culture has taught you that you can't be trusted with yummy foods, so you cannot trust your body and yourself. The normal body changes you begin to experience in midlife bring up *even more* fear and anxiety about your body no longer being in your control. Perimenopause and menopause add another layer to your vulnerability to diet/wellness and anti-aging messages. Again, this is not your fault.

Checking in

Time for a break. Facing how diet/wellness culture is embedded in your life and affects your relationship with your body is uncomfortable and potentially triggering.

Check in with yourself and notice how you are feeling. Soften your gaze, close your eyes, notice where you are making contact with the earth, and scan your body for any places you may be holding and bracing. Can you soften these places and offer yourself care and compassion in any manner that supports you? Be kind to yourself in this moment.

Anti-aging and diet culture—midlife women in the crosshairs

The upheaval you feel in midlife may create a longing for some sense of control, which takes root in your relationship with your body. There is a great deal of pressure to control your body in midlife+. It's understandable if you feel that you "should" be strict with your eating and exercise.

Besides health fears and concerns, why are you *more* vulnerable to diet and wellness culture as you age? Youth is highly valued, and as you get older, you feel less relevant, per the body hierarchy. You may feel less visible and pushed to the margins. Our culture's body hierarchy places a higher value on thin, fit, and able bodies, while bodies that are larger and less able have a lower value. You actually protect yourself from the loss of social currency if your older body is thin and fit/able (or at least perceived as working toward the ideal).

Social media is full of praise for older bodies doing superhuman things. I get it! It can feel "inspiring" to see stories of people in their 80s and 90s running races, lifting weights, and contorting their bodies into yoga shapes. And, understandably, you want to maintain your ability to function as you age. These messages make you feel like you are doing this aging thing "right" if you push yourself harder.

How does this strong narrative about thinness and fitness affect you as you age? Likely, this body story contributes to the pressure you feel to make your body your project. This pressure encourages a more disordered way of eating and exercising to achieve a body that gets attention, is valued, and belongs.

Meanwhile, you hear nothing about the threat this poses to your mental health. You hear nothing about the struggle of relapsing into disordered relationships with your body, eating, and movement. You hear nothing about the emotional burden of body shame.

To further complicate your experience, our culture normalizes and praises restriction and more intense exercise, so it is hard to recognize that you may be slipping into an unhealthy relationship with these thoughts and behaviors until you are in trouble. **Midlife+ culture normalizes disordered eating**.

Eating disorders in midlife

Disordered eating and exercise obsession are well-kept secrets for women in midlife and older. It might look like chronically "being careful" or skipping meals, planning your life around your exercise routine, or constantly trying the next fad diet. My clients tell me they feel stuck in their disordered thoughts and habits and very alone with their secrets. Comments by their loved ones, their healthcare providers, and even strangers on social media praising their thinness and fitness keep them trapped in their disorder. The body changes that accompany perimenopause and menopause may make you ramp up your efforts to control your body even more. When others affirm you for what they perceive as self-control and discipline, you double down on restriction and exercise.

Notes from an expert

Margo Maine, PhD, FAED, CEDS, therapist with over 40 years of experience treating eating disorders and body image issues, and the author of *Pursuing Perfection: Eating Disorders, Body Myths, and Women at Midlife and Beyond*:

> I continue to present on the topic of menopause, midlife, and eating disorders. There's very little new research to discuss. It's really, really just frustrating to me that it seems we don't care about older women. But there is increasing pressure to appear thin and young. There's a new term in the plastic surgery world called the "Glamma" instead of "Grandma," and the kind of plastic surgery you would do for an older woman to remove signs of aging. Along with the pressure to be thin. The message is if you have to get old, you've got to do it in a thin body.
>
> We put women out to pasture as they age.

The changes and losses accompanying midlife in work and romance may also contribute to your drive toward thinness and fitness. You may feel more interesting and attractive in a competitive and ageist workplace. Divorces increase during midlife. Entering the dating scene after divorce or widowhood increases your vulnerability to diet culture. For some, an "empty nest" is a big change and can be a stressful event, scrambling your identity in real ways.

If you've struggled with an eating disorder previously, periods of transition create a higher risk for relapse. While midlife can be exciting and adventurous, a new chapter invites the unknown into your life, creating vulnerability. Returning to the security of the familiar patterns of chronic dieting, over-exercising, or disordered eating can be a very slippery slope.

Please be aware: You can't tell someone has an eating disorder by looking at them. Thinness is *not* common for all eating disorders. As a matter of fact, only 6 percent of those diagnosed with an eating disorder are medically underweight. You cannot tell by looking at someone that they have an eating disorder because eating disorders are thought disorders.

Restricting, following food rules, and bingeing are common for the majority of eating disorders. So, eating disorders are perpetuated by diet/wellness culture. Yes, wellness. This is one of the reasons why wellness culture is especially sneaky and potentially dangerous.

What's wrong with wellness?

You've probably noticed that I tend to say diet/wellness culture rather than only diet culture. So here's why that is:

> "Wellness culture is a set of values that equate wellness with moral goodness and posits certain behaviors—and a certain type of body—as the path to achieving that supposed rectitude. Wellness culture overlaps with diet culture as a system of beliefs that regards thinness, muscularity, and particular body shapes as markers of health and moral virtue; promotes weight loss and body reshaping as a means

of attaining higher status; demonizes certain foods and food groups while elevating others; and oppresses people who don't match its supposed picture of health."

Christy Harrison, RD, The Wellness Trap

Slowly but surely, the word is getting out that "diets don't work." A few years ago, weight loss programs and plans began to lose money and quickly moved to rebrand themselves with the words "wellness" and "lifestyle." It's all semantics, though. Regardless of the vocabulary switcharoo, wellness culture is still quietly upholding the thin ideal. The undercurrent of weight loss and preferred thinness remains underneath the surface. I like to say that it is the same bullshit with glitter on top.

To be clear, the damaging hallmarks of dieting remain within wellness programs: food dichotomies—good and bad food choices, all-or-nothing thinking, guilt, and shame. The ubiquitous profitability of a wide-ranging wellness culture, which includes multi-level marketing schemes and social media "influencers," is very clear. The approach begins with loud fear-mongering, followed by a strong dose of pseudo-science, and ends with a sales pitch. Once you see this pattern, it becomes pretty obvious, and you see it everywhere! The changes in your body's shape, size, and functionality in midlife+ increase your vulnerability to these lies and promises.

The areas where Western medicine does not offer clear answers and support create a need for alternative therapies. It is well established that research in women's health is under-funded. We now have data that supports medical providers receiving little education about perimenopause, menopause, and post-menopause. If you are like most women, you are dis-appointed in finding providers who help you understand your midlife body and how to best care for it. It's no surprise that you seek help beyond conventional medical providers. This disappointment and desperation again create vulnerability to seeking care from the wellness industry.

Menopause as big business

There is a not-so-thinly veiled overlap between industries touting anti-aging products and those claiming to support women through menopause. With headlines like "Welcome To The Menopause Gold Rush," accompanied by an image of nude Gwyneth Paltrow covered in gold, it is easy to see the vultures circling. I am regularly contacted by companies that want me to endorse products and supplements touted to help women "balance their hormones" and "get their lives back on track." The sense that women are desperate to "fix" their aging bodies opens the door to capitalism at its worst, and it's infuriating.

While I am thrilled that we are finally talking seriously about perimenopause, menopause, and women's health, we need to recognize the opening this creates for diet/wellness culture to sell us solutions to problems they created. If you've been making your way to recovery from disordered eating or chronic dieting, it feels like diet/wellness rules are entering from an unsuspected side door of sorts.

The Lancet published a series of papers discussing the complicated topic of the "medicalization" of menopause in March 2024. *The Lancet* authors cited concern that women are being "targeted by a growing menopause industry that is eager to capitalize on their anxieties and cite evidence that for most women, menopause symptoms are not severe." Of course, if your symptoms are making your life difficult then that's all that matters.

During this complex and complicated time of transition, many companies have a commercial interest in portraying menopause, and your menopausal body, as a "problem," maybe even a "medical problem." This stance leaves you to parse through an overwhelming amount of information to find what is helpful for you and your unique body. How do you separate the hype from what's real? First, listen to your instincts. The menopause treatments being sold to us perpetuate a lot of negative feelings. Think about whether you really want to *own* these negative feelings. Could you tune into your own self instead?

This book is all about mending your relationship with your body so you can reclaim your ability to trust yourself. Remember: *You are the expert of you—it's time to listen to the expert.* It might take time and it will take work, but you will be more able to trust what your body is telling you.

In a culture where you feel valued for your appearance, coupled with a narrow beauty ideal lifting up youth and thinness above all else, it certainly makes sense that an event that signals the loss of your value feels like a problem. While I encourage you to choose what supports your well-being during menopause, I also advise considering the role our cultural messages play in your negative feelings about yourself in this chapter of your life.

Here's a story that you may relate to. It shows how easy it is to feel stuck in the anti-aging and diet/wellness mess as you age.

Barb's story

Barb led an active childhood. She played several sports and did not really think about what she ate. Why would she? Her mom went through cycles of dieting and was a sporadic Weight Watchers member, but Barb felt strong and confident in her body all the way through high school.

For her first few years of college, Barb remained active but didn't play any formal sports. But in her junior year, she went home for the holidays, and, for the first time, her family commented on her weight gain. Ashamed, Barb resolved to lose weight after New Years and signed up for WW, like her mother. Also on her mom's advice, Barb started a food journal.

And so Barb's history of weight cycling began. She ditched WW in her 30s for more restrictive diet plans, which only piled on restrictions as Barb entered perimenopause and menopause and started to feel her body was out of control.

I met Barb when she was 62, after she recently stopped dieting following her last very restrictive diet plan.

In our first session, after I asked her what brought her to me, she said, "I'm depleted, exhausted, and obsessive. I can't sleep. I think about food *all the time*." She sighed. "I just can't do it anymore. Part of me wants to start another diet, but I'm so tired of counting and calculating every bite I take. I want to put dieting behind me."

I wanted to do a happy dance and shout "Hell yeah!" but I refrained. Instead, I told her, "I fully support your decision. It's such a hard one to make because diet culture makes us feel like *we* are the failure, when really diets have a 95% failure rate."

Barb nodded. "The only time I didn't weight cycle was when I was pregnant, but afterwards it felt like I had to get my body back, you know? And I'd start a new diet."

We dug deeper into the reasons that kept Barb rethinking hopping back on that diet train.

"I'm just worried I don't *look fit* anymore," Barb added. "What if people don't think I'm healthy because I keep gaining weight?"

She felt she was losing her identity.

Like Barb, many people think you can look at someone and know if they are healthy and fit based on their size. But this is completely false. I once had a client who couldn't buy clothing in local shops, but she could ride her bike from our town to the closest mountain top and back. Plenty of people with thin or straight-sized bodies are no where close to her level of fitness.

It helps to do this myth-busting and also to acknowledge this is a real loss that stirs up all of the feelings that come with grief.

On the more positive side, this is also a great time to step back and reflect on your identity and values. How do you want to spend your time and energy? How do you want to feel? What do you want growing older to look like? What do you want your children (if you have them) to witness and remember about you?

What about you? What if you want to free yourself from this mess?

Finding your sweet spot

First of all, like I told Barb, I support you. Nourishing and caring for your body as you step away from anti-aging and diet/wellness culture messages is courageous. This alternative path can also be a way of connecting with your internal compass and feeling empowered to follow your instincts. Part 2 will lead you to make choices guided by your unique body wisdom that prioritize your vitality and well-being without focusing on controlling your body's size and shape.

But before we get into the mending process, let's take a closer look at how the conversation about exercise and fitness is another important part of how our relationships with our bodies have gotten twisted up in diet/wellness and anti-aging/longevity messages.

3

Exercise dogma—never enough

One of my favorite things is playing with my grandchildren, or any children, really. I absolutely adore how carefree they are as they spin and skip and climb and dance, oblivious to any worry about what their bodies look like. It reminds me that our bodies can be passports to our vitality and joy! Movement can be natural, playful, and pleasurable. Yet, an easy and enjoyable relationship with movement is out of reach for many of us. When and how did your relationship with moving your body get complicated? Or maybe this easy relationship with movement was not your starting place.

Some of us are born attuned to our bodies, with our "default factory settings" wired for an innate desire to move, but this isn't the case for everyone. We experience varying degrees of connection and ease with our bodies. As with most things, there is no right and wrong way to feel about moving our bodies. Perhaps you are highly sensitive, making movement uncomfortable for you. Maybe you grew up with less access to space to run and play, or it wasn't safe. Or maybe you experienced trauma, so you no longer feel safe in your body, complicating your relationship with movement. Or maybe you simply prefer the company of books and quiet and are attracted to being still. We are all beautifully unique.

For most of us, something happened that made us start worrying over and judging our moving bodies. We became conscious of our bodies and what others think of them. Your Body Story that you wrote in Chapter 1 may have included this experience. If your family or friends valued appearance, performance, or fitness, their opinions about your body may have entered your life early and frequently. After these experiences and comments, it's no wonder you started to see your body's movement with judgment, criticism, or feel shame.

If your relationship with eating and your body is complicated, your relationship with movement is likely also complex. This chapter will explore how external forces have likely disrupted your relationship with moving your body. I rarely use the word "exercise" because it can be triggering. I am more comfortable talking about moving our bodies with the more descriptive and neutral term, movement. Exercise is moving your body as part of a transaction, typically with an expectation that you are fixing your body or managing it somehow.

Before we begin, check in with yourself using one of the grounding or body scan practices in earlier chapters. Then, grab your journal and answer these questions:

- How did you feel about playing as a child?
- What were your favorite ways to play?

What specific memories come to mind? Describe these memories in as much detail as possible. What do you feel, smell, hear, and see as you remember playing?

- Do you have any memories of negative experiences associated with playing at home, school, dance, or sports? Describe these memories in as much detail as possible. What do you feel, smell, hear, and see as you remember playing?
- Note: *It is okay to pass if this does not feel safe for you.*
- Were there any particular comments from teachers, coaches, family, or friends that affect how you feel about moving your body?
- Describe your current relationship with movement. Have there been chapters of your life where this relationship was easier? More complicated?

Let's unpack how your relationship with movement may have become complicated. Please be assured that you will learn ways to repair this rupture as we discuss reclaiming attuned and playful movement in Chapter 6.

Becoming self-conscious

I am curious about the moment when you shifted from feeling easily connected to your body, or embodied, to becoming "self-conscious." When did you begin looking at your body with judgment? Hopefully answering the questions above increased your awareness of how and when this happened to you.

A client once described her experience when she was in the second grade. Her best friend started playing more with other girls in the neighborhood and stopped playing with her. Her mother encouraged her to approach her friend and ask why she didn't want to play with her anymore. She was shocked, hurt, and full of shame when her friend told her that she didn't want to play with her anymore because she was chubby. Another client told me about being an "early bloomer" and starting to develop breasts when she was nine years old. She was teased about her body changes and was abruptly thrown into consciousness and shame about her body. She described feeling suddenly acutely aware of her body and as though she couldn't run and play like she did before.

These are great descriptions of the subtle, and not so subtle, shift when we began to look at our bodies because we noticed others looking at our bodies. You may be an outlier and feel comfortable with how moving your body feels. However, my personal and professional experiences demonstrate that body judgment is a part of our daily lives in little ways and not so little ways. When we look at our bodies and how we move and perform, we compare and criticize, likely followed by feelings of self-doubt and shame.

If you are fortunate, there was once a time when moving your body meant feeling connected to your body, playful, and pleasurable. Becoming self-conscious about your body ruptures this connection. Niva Piran, author of *Handbook of Positive Body Image and Embodiment: Constructs, Protective Factors, and Interventions*, says: "Post-puberty, joyful immersion and agency in physical activities are commonly replaced by compulsive, often joyless physical activities aimed at body alterations—such as weight loss or body sculpting—anchored in experiences of deficiency rather than agency."

Most of us have experienced this at different times and stages in our lives. You are fortunate if you made it to puberty before this happened to you. Certainly, puberty is when we experience sudden and significant body changes. This may create feelings of insecurity and discomfort in our bodies. Our body size, shape, and performance may have been judged. One of the most difficult movement memories my clients in the US have in common is the President's Physical Fitness Test.

President's Physical Fitness Test

If you were lucky enough to escape this annual ritual of childhood public humiliation, here is a brief description of the President's Physical Fitness Test. Beginning in 1958, every class in the US public schools was given a battery of tests, such as pull-ups, sit-ups, a reach test, a one-mile run and relays, rope climbs, throws, and jumps. At the end, each kid received a publicly stated score. Despite a lack of critical evidence, adults widely accepted this was for our own good.

If that wasn't enough embarrassment, in the 1980s, an updated version of the test added weighing, testing body composition, and calculating the BMI, which moved the test toward the moral panic we remember from the 1980s and 90s about "pediatric ob*sity." Overall, this test did little to promote movement but did attach a traumatic experience to physical activity and, for many, contributed to body shame.

Who thought it was a good idea to test kids with activities most kids never engaged in, I might add, with their peers in a school setting? What could possibly go wrong? Insert massive eye roll. The *Maintenance Phase* podcast did a fabulous job researching the history of the President's Physical Fitness Test. It is worth a listen!

So many of us have painful memories of this test, and it likely affected how you felt about your body and movement. You may carry the same feeling to this day! And while we're on the subject of ill-advised campaigns to encourage movement, let's talk about 10,000 steps, shall we?

The myth of 10,000 steps

The concept that walking 10,000 steps each day will improve your overall health is part of our modern-day wellness lexicon. This hugely successful marketing campaign was launched ahead of the 1964 Tokyo Olympics. You may be surprised to learn, as I certainly was, that marketers chose this number because the Japanese character for 10,000 resembles a person walking, and the idea caught on. This number of steps is related to no actual data. Yup, you heard me correctly. The number of steps itself is not supported by any solid scientific foundation. Mind-blowing!

Today, this concept goes unquestioned and is embedded in our daily lives through the products we frequently use, such as our smartwatches and smartphones.

Numerous studies show that getting more movement supports your well-being on multiple levels. There is no debate about that. However, where is the tipping point at which we no longer benefit from the additional effort? This is a great question, and the answer depends on who you ask. I've read many studies offering varying answers. It is truly a moving target. When are we sacrificing other aspects of our health, creative projects, relationships, etc., when we choose to move for a longer period of time or more frequently?

Overall, we are bio-psycho-social animals who become more unique as we age. No population-based answer to this question is helpful to us as individuals. These "exercise recommendations" contribute to the "shoulds" we hear about moving our bodies, which can easily feel like added pressure and become another item on our long to-do list or another stressor.

When we talk about counting our steps, we must consider how we track our bodies' movements. So, what about those tracking devices? Do they really support our well-being?

Fitness trackers

I vividly remember the first time I heard about a fitness tracker. I was a consultant for a research project in the 1990s, and the exercise physiologist was wearing one and wanted to use it in the study we were discussing. She was so excited! I was a little bit horrified. Since then, my concern has only amplified after working with countless clients whose experience with these gadgets contributed to their disordered relationship with movement and their bodies.

Do you feel like you "should" keep going to match the number on your device with a goal from an external source? Or do you stop your movement for the day because your body says you're done? When you no longer tune into how your body feels because you rely on guidance from a gadget, you can miss important information from the ultimate source of wisdom. You miss potential cues for rest or a desire for more movement. More than anything, you no longer feel curious about how you are feeling and what you are sensing because you are watching the readout of a device.

In my experience with clients, any behavior that can be reduced to a number can trigger obsessive-compulsive thoughts and behaviors and, ultimately, guilt and shame. Diet and fitness culture thrive on reducing our experience to a measurable achievement, and fitness trackers hook us into this mindset. The seduction feels like you are trying to win at a game and continue to beat your "personal best," aka personal record. These external gadgets make it nearly impossible to be present for your experience.

According to Anna Lembke, a professor of psychiatry and behavioral sciences at Stanford University and the author of *Dopamine Nation: Finding Balance in the Age of Indulgence*:

> "These technologies have, in essence, drug-ified even exercise. You may think, 'A wearable device that keeps track of my actions couldn't possibly be bad because it's just a watch, and I'm just, for example, monitoring my heart rate, which is about my physical wellness.' But in fact, we very much can become compulsively fixated on these wearable devices—in a way that is akin to addiction."

In modern life, we tend to use devices to measure our experience rather than pausing and checking in with ourselves. Social media further complicates our relationship to moving our bodies. How do you feel when you scroll through social media posts about fitness inspiration or "fitspo" from fitness influencers?

Fitness influencers

In the early days of my career, I sought out exercise physiologists for my clients who were interested in their support. Mind you, this was before the internet was a thing! So, getting to know the credentials and philosophies of the trainers I referred to was as simple as making a call, visiting a gym, or making a date to grab a cup of coffee. We developed a relationship.

Now, my clients are exposed to a multitude of content on social media by "fitness influencers." As of 2023, more than 50,000 fitness influencers were on social media. A study published in *BMC Public Health* (Curtis et al., 2023) stated: "Nearly two-thirds of the 100 most popular fitness influencers lacked sound advice or posted messages that could negatively affect people's mental and physical health by promoting exercise as a tool to become skinnier." No question that fitness culture is deeply entangled with diet culture.

Growing evidence supports that exposure to images encouraging a specific physique correlates with decreased body satisfaction and mood. Not surprisingly, it has also been linked to disordered eating.

Fitness influencers often portray an idealized version of health and fitness. Their perfectly curated posts can set unrealistic standards for us, leading to feelings of inadequacy and pressure to meet those unattainable goals. Often, these influencers live with a degree of privilege with fewer demands on their time and access to resources, such as personal trainers, nutritionists, and professional photographers, that the average person doesn't. I can't overstate that genetics plays a major role in appearance, including body size and composition. Yet, influencers' messages lead you to believe that your body's size and shape are within your control—if you just work physically hard enough and have enough mental discipline.

With countless fitness influencers sharing various workout routines, diet plans, and health tips, it can be overwhelming to sift through all the information. Many of my clients say they're overwhelmed, lost, and confused by conflicting advice, making it hard to know which path to follow for their well-being. The constant exposure to seemingly perfect bodies and lifestyles trips you into the comparison trap, which contributes to anxiety and depression.

Remember, we are all unique, and bodies come in all shapes and sizes. There is no such thing as a "good" and "bad" body! Social media often presents a highlight reel rather than reality, including professional lighting, camera angles, photoshopped images, and filters.

It is challenging to discern which accounts are helpful and which are harmful. I am extremely cautious about making recommendations, but I trust some movement professionals. I've included them in the Resources section. Otherwise, trust your instincts! Unfollow or mute accounts that leave you feeling like you are not enough, negatively about aging, or critical of your body. This gets even trickier when looking for accounts with an age-affirming attitude about movement.

What about pro-aging fitness influencers?

Since I started my research on evidence-based ways to support the well-being of those in midlife and older, recommendations for physical activity in midlife+ have increased in intensity. As of this writing, the fitness influencers focusing on aging "well" recommend:

- Strength training, which has escalated into "heavy lifting"
- Endurance activity, which has escalated into "HIIT workouts."

In general, HIIT workouts are high-intensity interval training that alternates periods of high-intensity exercise with brief rest periods. There is ongoing debate about the specifics of these periods.

Don't get me wrong, I encourage you to engage in movement as long as you are able and interested and do it at a level that benefits your well-being. Of course this can include strength training and endurance activities. However, if you keep up with the trendy "recommendations" for moving your body as you age, this may leave you feeling like what you are doing is never enough. If you've had a disordered relationship with your body, movement, or eating in your life, this tone of "never enough" can be triggering and potentially harmful.

Sadly, most fitness influencers promote anti-aging and weight-loss products and services, often blurring the line between genuine advice and marketing. This commercialization can make it difficult to discern authentic recommendations from paid promotions. It's not easy to separate the false hype from what is truly helpful.

Since we become more heterogeneous the longer we live, generalized advice from a fitness influencer may not be suitable for you. One-size-fits-all regimens are potentially risky and can sometimes lead to injury or adverse health effects. If you want support for movement, you are better off leaving social media and finding a professional to help you create personalized movement plans tailored to your body and interests. One or two sessions may be enough to answer your questions.

My greatest concern is how easily you can get caught up in diet culture when you start thinking about movement. In other words, one of my goals for this book is to help you consistently adopt a growing awareness of the damage fitness and diet culture are doing.

Entangled with diet culture/weight loss (calories in/calories out)

Diet culture tells you to move your body primarily to burn calories and lose weight. While there are numerous health benefits and potential for play and pleasure, focusing on moving your body to control your weight destroys the intrinsic joys and whole-person benefits of physical activity, such as:

- Improving mental health
- Increasing strength
- Enhancing mobility
- Maintaining metabolic, brain, and heart health
- Protecting muscle and bone mass

- Maintaining flexibility and balance
- Promoting overall well-being.

Diet culture often perpetuates a specific definition of beauty and health, emphasizing youth, thinness, and specific body shapes. When you move primarily to achieve this narrowly defined look rather than to connect to your body and have fun, this harms your body image and mental health. It can also result in issues like body dysmorphia and shame.

With this narrow focus, who gets left out? Fitness culture entangled with diet culture often excludes bodies of diverse size and shape, age, gender identity, color, culture, abilities, and movement capacity, creating an unwelcoming environment for many people. This lack of diversity may discourage you from engaging in movement if you don't see yourself represented or feel judged because your body doesn't conform to that narrow standard.

Diet culture can lead you to think movement is used to "earn" food or "make up for" eating, leading to guilt and shame. This unhealthy relationship with movement can result in stress, anxiety, and even a disordered relationship with your body, eating, and movement.

Overemphasizing weight loss as the primary reason for moving your body can undermine other important aspects of movement, such as improving your mood or supporting your muscle mass and bone health. Keeping your focus narrowed to only controlling your body's size and shape can lead to an unbalanced relationship with movement, such as exercise resistance or addiction.

Understanding exercise resistance

If exercise was a part of your disordered eating in the past, a wise and protective part of you understands that and creates a resistance to movement. You may have forced yourself to follow rigid exercise rules, like working out despite being tired, sick, or even injured. You may have pushed yourself to participate in exercise programs you did not enjoy. Therefore, there may be a part of you that is not sure engaging in movement again is in your best interest, leaving you resistant to engaging in movement.

If this resonates, you are not alone. This is a common theme in my work with clients healing their relationship with their bodies. Many people develop negative associations with movement because it has been framed as a chore or punishment rather than something to look forward to. A fitness culture entangled with diet culture creates societal pressures, and we are all familiar with thin ideals that persist here, too. This pressure turns exercise into a dreaded obligation rather than a way to play and care for your body.

It is more common than not to have traumatic experiences related to moving your body, such as being bullied or body-shamed at a gym or yoga studio or, in general, while involved in physical activity. I've had countless clients tell me about being harassed about their bodies when they were out for a walk or a run or in gym class in school.

Sometimes, people are unaware of their anti-fat bias and will comment "good for you" only to the person in a larger body, causing harm and body shame. It is not easy to join a class or go to a gym or studio when you are concerned about comments from others. If this has happened to you, give yourself some compassion and understanding about resistance to exercise.

Barriers to movement can also include a lack of time, energy, resources, or access to safe and welcoming exercise environments. Disabilities or chronic health conditions can also contribute to resistance. Resistance is real, usualy complicated, and nothing to be ashamed of.

If you were pressured to move your body primarily as a tool for weight loss or sculpting your body, and you didn't get those results, it's understandable that you are resistant to begin again. Sometimes, you just aren't feeling up to it, and that's okay, too. Be gentle with yourself. Beating yourself up for your resistance will only contribute to your feeling stuck.

If you believe that aging means you are no longer capable of being strong, flexible, or vital, you are less likely to engage in activity. Internalized ageism can be a self-fulfilling prophecy—what you believe about aging will be your experience. Alternatively, there is also a possibility that your relationship with movement may become unhealthy when it feels compulsive or addictive.

Understanding exercise "addiction"

Exercise addiction, also known as compulsive exercise or exercise dependence, is a condition where you engage in physical activity to the point where it negatively impacts your physical and mental health, social life, and overall well-being. Exercise addiction is characterized by an obsession with physical activity, where you feel compelled to exercise and prioritize it over other aspects of your life. Symptoms can include:

- Exercising despite injury or illness
- Experiencing withdrawal symptoms (e.g., anxiety, irritability) when unable to exercise
- Neglecting yourself, others or your responsibilities in favor of being active
- Continuously increasing the amount of movement to achieve the same effects.

Diet culture often promotes the idea that more exercise is always better and glorifies extreme dedication to fitness, which can lead to an unbalanced relationship with movement. The physiological changes of aging, such as loss of muscle mass, changes in hormones, and your metabolism, may cause your body to shift in size, shape, and composition. Societal pressures to maintain a youthful, thin, and fit body may drive you towards adding more intense, more frequent, or more types of movement. This can lead to an exercise compulsion as you seek to control the changes in your aging body.

You may also find accepting the body changes and losses you experience in midlife and beyond a significant challenge.

Most of us experience multiple losses in midlife, which causes varying experiences of grief. It is fairly common to experience a divorce, your children leave home, you feel passed over at work, you lose a friend, or you experience a combination of these events. Compulsive exercise may be your way to cope with emotional discomfort, loss, and the understandable, unsettled feelings of transition. This way of using movement to help you deal with life is sneaky and may lead to a harmful cycle of dependency on movement.

While moving your body is generally beneficial, excessive movement can lead to serious consequences to your well-being, including:

- Increased risk of injuries, such as stress fractures and tendonitis
- Weakened immune system
- Further complicating hormonal changes
- Chronic fatigue
- Burnout
- Contributing to an eating disorder
- Disrupting social relationships and work performance
- Mental health issues like anxiety and depression.

Another way your relationship with movement may become disruptive and more like a have-to than a want-to is by associating activity with longevity or "aging backward." At first glance, moving your body to age "well" seems like a great idea. Let's take a look at the shadow side of movement for longevity.

The problems with moving for longevity

While regular movement is linked to increased lifespan, an excessive focus on activity solely for longevity can overshadow the importance of quality of life. Prioritizing activities you believe are optimal for lifespan extension over those you genuinely enjoy reduces your capacity for playfulness, pleasure, and satisfaction. Movement motivated by fear takes the fun out of activities.

Intensive regimens that "maximize longevity" can lead to overtraining. This can cause physical injuries, fatigue, and mental burnout, ultimately counteracting the benefits of movement and possibly contributing to stress, anxiety, and problems with sleep.

Constantly striving for longevity through movement adds stress to your life and worsens perfectionistic tendencies. If you approach your movement with rigidity and an excessive drive to do everything right, your activity will consume significant time and energy, potentially isolating you from social activities and relationships that are just as important for a long and fulfilling life. Striking the balance can be a real challenge.

Overemphasis on lifespan extension through movement can lead to physical and mental health issues, social isolation, and, counter-intuitively, a diminished quality of life. If this resonates with you, don't add worrying about overdoing your movement to your stress list. Chapter 6 will discuss ways to create a more balanced and healthy relationship with movement.

Another aspect of this shadow side of movement for aging well is the focus on "super-agers."

Super-agers

"Guinness World Record for longest plank time broken by a 58-year-old woman."

"87-year-old man is the oldest person to complete an Ironman World Championship."

"64-year-old woman is the first to swim the Florida Strait between Florida and Cuba."

Headlines like these are inspiring, right? Sure, but there are some problems with this phenomenon. "Super-agers" maintain high cognitive and physical function well into older ages. The nature of a bell curve is to have outliers. But what happens when we primarily hear stories about these outliers and rarely hear about the experiences of those in the majority or the middle of the bell curve? Here are some ways these sensationalized stories about the "super-aging" outliers may complicate your relationship with movement.

Societal pressure and ageism

How do you respond to these headlines celebrating super-agers? I remember seeing the story about the woman who broke the record for holding a plank position. I compared myself and timed how long I could hold a plank (while Netflix was on pause). Guess what? I was nowhere close, of course. I wrote about this in my newsletter and received many responses from women who resonated with feeling insufficient, which is exactly how I felt. I'm not taking anything away from the woman who broke the record! I'm concerned about the media frenzy around her doing so. The loud media coverage of stories about super-agers can inadvertently contribute to ageism by reinforcing that only those who defy the typical aging process are valuable or worthy of admiration. This can create more pressure to conform to these ideals, leading to age-related stigma for those who experience aging differently.

Focusing too much on super-agers can overshadow your experiences and needs. Most of us will not achieve super-ager status, and this narrative can marginalize the majority of us who are aging in more typical ways. Genetics, access to training facilities, time, financial and social support, and sheer luck of having an able body and energy for training combine to influence the ability to become a super-ager.

The popular film *Nyad*, based on the true story of Diane Nyad's journey to be the first to swim the Florida Strait, perfectly illustrates the resources and support she needed for this feat.

Of course, she worked intensely hard and needed to endure pain and hardship to do this. And I think this film perfectly illustrates the shadow side along with the celebration. It is helpful to notice how easily we lift up this story as a success with little curiosity about her and her team's well-being.

Most factors that allow a super-ager to engage in what looks to be super-human are beyond your control, which means not everyone has the same potential to achieve super-ager status, regardless of their efforts. The portrayals of super-agers in the media typically oversimplify and neglect to report on the potential negative consequences.

While the concept of super-agers is inspiring, it is crucial to approach it with a balanced perspective. Another concerning aspect of what we are typically told about movement and aging lives in the underbelly of ableism.

Ableism

Ableism, which involves discrimination and social prejudice against people with disabilities, manifests in various ways within fitness culture and impacts our potential ability to engage in and benefit from physical activity. Ageism and ableism are often linked, so here is a heads-up to stay curious.

Ableism is a sneaky and subtle issue that can create barriers and exclude some of us. The fitness space for midlife and older people perpetuates assumptions and stereotypes about aging and physical ability. I hope this is changing. The sources listed in the Resources section are change-makers in the fitness world.

As we've discussed, fitness programs and advice often focus on high-intensity activities that may not be accessible to everyone, especially those with less capacity. This can create an environment where only certain types of bodies and abilities are valued. The obvious aspect of this consideration is that fitness facilities and programs are not designed with individuals with disabilities in mind. Lack of accessible equipment, spaces, and classes tailored to varying levels of mobility can exclude many people from participating in fitness activities.

The more subtle aspect of this issue is that our culture is quick to applaud and celebrate the super-agers. Simultaneously, we often hold negative views about aging with disability or less capacity, seeing these bodies as problems to be fixed rather than natural variations of the human experience. This can make us feel unwelcome or embarrassed to participate in fitness activities, fearing judgment or pity.

We are so accustomed to our ableist fitness culture, which emphasizes "fixing" bodies through exercise and suggests that fitness should eliminate the signs of aging or disability. This can create unrealistic expectations and pressure on us to conform to these standards rather than embracing our unique bodies and abilities. Ableism in fitness for aging is a pervasive issue that can limit our interest in participating and enjoying moving our bodies.

Judy's story

Judy was 43 when she contacted me about working with her. Her spirit was bright, and she had an exceptionally sunny disposition. I am usually grateful for the honor of doing this work and, sometimes, deep gratitude washes over me when I begin to work with someone. Judy was one of those clients.

When Judy was eight years old, she was diagnosed with diabetes mellitus type I. She dedicated her life's work to those who shared her experience, working as a registered dietitian and a certified diabetes educator. She contacted me as perimenopause was beginning to complicate her life, throwing a surprising wrench in her ability to control her body.

Her relationship with movement played a primary role in her identity, alongside her stellar "control" of her blood sugar. She involved herself with several different activities every day, was not able to sit still for any period of time, and was starting to experience "over-use" injuries in her 40s. She confided in me that her partner and friends expressed frustration with her tendency to run late or "flake" when she planned to get together. She knew it was because she prioritized exercise over her relationships.

Several months into our work together, Judy became more aware of her compulsion to move her body and how deeply she depended on movement to cope with or avoid uncomfortable feelings. Her need to calculate her eating to manage her blood sugar was also clear. Of course, she experienced benefits and received much praise for controlling her body size, shape, and blood sugar. The more we discussed her relationship with her body, the more she was aware of her disconnection and disembodiment. She was already working with a therapist, so these new insights became a new focus for her work in therapy.

The more I offered small challenges to develop a caring relationship with her body rather than a problem she felt determined to "be on top of," the more she became aware of how entrenched this way of thinking was for her. Experimenting with a rest day was difficult and often impossible. Trying to take a day off from her movement routine made her anxious, irritable, and irrationally guilty. It was challenging for her to eat on rest days.

Judy was also beginning to see that a part of her was really tired of her movement regimen. When challenged to begin to notice how her body was feeling or notice her sensations, she expressed frustration and feeling lost. When encouraged to go play without tracking or numbers, she simply felt that type of movement "did not count."

Let's leave Judy's story here for now. We will return to how she mends her relationship with her body in Chapter 6.

Journaling exercise

Take a moment to set the book aside and check in with yourself again. You know the drill.

Now that we've explored experiences and beliefs that may have complicated your relationship with movement, please journal about your response to a question from early in this chapter:

- How would you describe your current relationship with movement? Have there been chapters of your life where this relationship was easier? More complicated?

- Are you recognizing some resistance to moving your body? What does that look like and feel like in your life?
- Are you concerned that your relationship with movement veers into a compulsion? What does that look like and feel like in your life?
- Can you understand the circumstances that have contributed to your relationship with movement? Write about this part of your life story.
- Can you feel compassion for yourself now that you understand more about what brought you here?
- Do you want to address or change things about your relationship with moving your body?
- What would these changes look like? Please permit yourself to move slowly and with kindness toward yourself. Small steps, please!

Mending the rupture

Okay, now that you've developed some awareness and insight into all of the ways your relationship may be complicated, please give yourself a break. The good news is that you are never too old or too late to mend your relationship with your body and how you care for yourself. In Chapter 6, we'll explore concepts and practices for healing the rupture you have with movement.

4

Ageism and body shame— a dysregulated nervous system

Sarah's story

Sarah was one of our group's kindest and, by far, the most calm and collected member. She consistently validated the feelings and experiences of her fellow participants. She was quick to share vulnerable stories about her struggles with body image and food judgment.

But today, she was fidgety, unable to get her hair just right, and clearly uncomfortable. Midway through our session, she anxiously reported that she had a story to tell us, asking if we were okay with her sharing it.

Of course, we were okay. We are all about having each other's backs.

It was about week six of our eight-week group program, so we already knew some of Sarah's back story. She experienced an eating disorder as a teenager and was hospitalized for treatment, which she described as traumatizing. As an adult, Sarah was in and out of her recovery. At this point in her life, in her early 50s, she was feeling pretty strong about her recovery, but menopause was messing with her body image, and she was beginning to think more about restrictive diets. Sarah found my work and decided to participate in my group coaching instead of starting another diet plan. She was exceptional in her excitement about what we were up to, saying that she was so tired of dieting, but she also felt committed to accepting the changes in her body, and I loved everything about that!

Three days ago, Sarah's office was celebrating several birthdays with doughnuts, and she decided to challenge her food fears by enjoying one. She was particularly elated by this choice and her success. Still carrying the last few bites of her doughnut in a napkin, she left the celebration and entered another office, where she met several women gathered around the mailboxes. One of the women eyed her treat and said, "Do you know how many calories are in that?!"

Sarah froze as the shame from eating the doughnut washed over her. Struck dumb, she could not find any words for a response in the face of her co-worker's food judgment and dashed out of the office, throwing away the last few bites of her doughnut on her way out.

In the privacy of her office, she experienced a full-blown panic attack—she had not had one in months! Their judgment triggered the criticism and shame of the eating disorder part of her, which dysregulated her nervous system. She took the next day off from work. This event happened three days before her telling of this story.

"I'm just now starting to feel like myself," she confessed to the group. "I was so surprised that something that seemed like such a small thing could undo me."

Sarah's story is not that uncommon. How we feel about our bodies translates to how safe we feel in our world. Many clients have told me that they feel less safe in the world when they gain weight or look older. Our ability to feel secure is directly related to the regulated or dysregulated state of our nervous systems and vice versa. Additionally, stress is a significant player in our well-being, especially as we age. So, we cannot talk about our relationships with our aging bodies without discussing the importance of regulating our nervous systems.

In this chapter, you'll learn some basics about your nervous system:

- What is dysregulation? And what does it feel like?
- The intersection of shame, body shame, and nervous system regulation.
- How does our culture's body hierarchy and systemic oppression affect your nervous system?
- What roles do weight stigma and ageism play in your nervous system regulation?
- What happens when you shift from seeing you as an individual as responsible to the systems you live in?

- We're going to dig into the relationship between white supremacy, patriarchy, diet culture, and the added layer of ageism.
- How might aging with body liberation affect your body shame and nervous system?

This chapter also offers journal prompts to explore your awareness of your nervous system, body shame, and the body hierarchy, along with practices for regulating your nervous system and invitations to use them. Let's begin with the basics.

Nervous system regulation basics

Your nervous system makes your body's world go round! It presides over everything that makes you human: your consciousness, thoughts, behaviors, and memories.

Your nervous system is a complicated and vast network of neurons whose most significant job is generating, moderating, and transmitting information between your body's parts. It regulates all your vital bodily functions (cardiac function, breathing, digestion) and allows you to experience your senses, thoughts, emotions, and movements. Your nervous system significantly contributes to whether you feel like you are having a good day or not—every day of your life.

More specifically, your nervous system is divided into two main parts.

Central nervous system (CNS)

Comprising your brain and spinal cord, the CNS controls the processing and sending of instructions. Your brain interprets sensory information and coordinates bodily functions, while the spinal cord acts as a pathway for messages between the brain and the rest of the body.

Peripheral nervous system (PNS)

Your PNS includes all the nerves outside your CNS. It further divides into:

- Somatic nervous system, which controls your voluntary movements by activating skeletal muscles
- Autonomic nervous system, which manages your involuntary functions like heart, digestion, and respiratory rate. The ANS has two main branches:
  o Sympathetic nervous system: This system prepares your body for "fight or flight, freeze, flop, or fawn/friend" responses to perceived threats (see below)
  o Parasympathetic nervous system: This system promotes "rest and digest" activities, helping your body relax, regulate, and restore.

A regulated nervous system supports your optimal well-being as you age

A regulated nervous system ensures your body adapts to changes in your environment so your body maintains homeostasis or balance. This includes regulating:

- Responses to stressors
- Sleep
- Appetite and digestion
- Mood management
- Focus and attention
- General functioning of all your bodily systems.

When you place too much stress on your nervous system, this creates dysregulation. Inadequate nutrition, chronic stress, genetic predisposition, environmental stress, systemic oppression, and menopause contribute to nervous system dysregulation. However, for the purposes of our conversation, we'll focus on the effects of diet and trauma on your nervous system.

Not meeting your body's energy needs, undereating, or restricting calorie and carbohydrate intake contributes to nervous system dysregulation. Your brain uses 20–25 percent of your calories and requires carbohydrates to function optimally. Deficiencies in certain essential nutrients for the proper functioning of the nervous system, such as B12 and omega-3 fatty acids, may also contribute to dysregulation. It's important to note that we are all unique and have diverse nutritional needs based on our medications, disease processes, histories, and genetics. We'll discuss nourishing your body more in the next chapter.

Traumatic events affect each of us and our nervous systems differently

There are many ways to define trauma. The one that best fits my professional and personal experience is one I learned in "Healing Trauma with The Body" training with beloved teachers, Michael Stone and Molly Boeder Harris: "*Trauma is a breach of one's protective barrier, either physical, mental, energetic, or spiritual.* The event or series of events that caused the trauma passes, but the body still believes it's under threat. This taxes all of the body's systems, and we begin to experience wide-ranging symptoms and imbalances that can become chronic."

What you and I experience as traumatic varies widely, so this definition encompasses a wide range of events and ordeals.

What does nervous system dysregulation feel like?

Nervous system dysregulation feels different for different people and is different for various situations. It can feel like you are stuck in overdrive or hypervigilance, shut down, or numbed out.

The "fight, flight, freeze, flop, and fawn/friend" responses are reactions to stress or perceived danger. They are part of your body's instinctual survival mechanisms, orchestrated by the nervous system. You are wired for survival, which shows up when you perceive a threat in the present moment or when your experience "triggers" stressors or threats your mind or body remembers from the past. These triggers evoke a strong emotional response because something reminds you of a past traumatic event.

You are probably familiar with the often-discussed trauma responses of fight, flight, or freeze. However, there are the additional responses flop, and fawn/friend. "Flop", is similar to "freeze" but your muscles go limp or you body becomes floppy in the face of a perceived threat, similar to freezing, potentially protecting you from the physical pain of what's happening to you. If you "fawn/friend" in the face of trauma, you "people-please" or seek to make friends as a protective response to your experiences in childhood or emotionally unhealthy relationships. You prioritize the needs of others before your own and use "toxic positivity" and only "look on the bright side," as a way to protect yourself from experiencing emotional pain, leaving you disconnected from your body and experience. This response often goes unnoticed or even affirmed.

When your nervous system is dysregulated, it can show up in physical, emotional, and cognitive symptoms.

Common physical symptoms include:

- Elevated or irregular heart rate
- Nausea or diarrhea
- Shortness of breath
- Sweating
- Problems with sleep
- Body curving inward, protective stance
- Tightness in your neck and shoulders or other muscle groups
- Chronic headaches.

Common emotional symptoms include:

- Anxiety or agitation
- Feeling overstimulated/overwhelmed

- Numbing, foggy, or swirling feeling
- Disconnection from your body and/or your environment
- Feeling frozen or "stuck"
- Feeling on edge
- Irritability or reactivity
- Depression or feeling shut down.

Common cognitive symptoms include:

- Difficulty focusing or concentrating
- Problems with memory.

This is not an exhaustive list, but includes the most common experiences. We all experience some of these symptoms sometimes, and that's okay. However, there is reason for concern and care if you experience more of these symptoms frequently or feel stuck there.

Nervous system dysregulation is your body's response to feeling unsafe. Sometimes, these responses make perfect sense. And sometimes, we are unaware of why we are bracing for a threat!

- How does your body feel when anticipating an appointment with your accountant or healthcare provider?
- Are there particular memories that bring your shoulders up to your ears, when you are gritting your teeth?
- Are there certain people who when you hear their voices or see their names pop up on your phone's screen, you can sense your body braces and you feel "on guard"?
- Do you know people who make you feel calm and relaxed when you are around them and are rarely a "headache"?

If you notice how you feel dysregulated in certain circumstances and not in others, this can tell you quite a bit about your life, relationships, and yourself—including how you feel about your body or how our culture perceives your body.

Nervous system dysregulation might be easier to understand through experience rather than reading about it. Here is a practice for when you realize that you are dysregulated.

Practice

The best practices that support you depend on whether you are in fight, flight, freeze, flop, or fawn/friend. The Resources section of this book offers a variety of practices you can experiment with to see what best meets your needs. One essential practice is a good old-fashioned body scan (because you may or may not know what you need in the moment).

Body scan practice

Body scans encourage and embody mindfulness. They also help ground and calm your body so you can connect and discern more about what is happening with you and what you might need.

Here's a guided body scan practice:

1 *Preparation*: Make your body as comfortable as possible. Lie down on your back, sit comfortably in a chair, or even stand if that's more comfortable for you. If you need to move, slowly walk around as you scan your body. Close your eyes or allow your gaze to soften and rest in front of you, whichever is most comfortable.

2 *If it is comfortable for you, focus on your breath*: Take a few deep breaths. Inhale deeply through your nose, and exhale slowly through your mouth. It may be helpful to exhale with a sigh. Notice the sensation of your breath entering and leaving your body. Allow your breathing to settle into a natural rhythm. Trust that your body knows how to breathe.
Note: *If focusing on your breath makes you uncomfortable or causes distress, skip this step and know you are not alone.*

3 *Start at your feet (unless you have chronic pain and concerns about your feet, such as neuropathy. In which case, begin at a place that feels more natural to you)*: Bring your attention to your feet. Notice any sensations there—warmth, coolness, tingling, pressure, or numbness. Don't judge the sensations; simply observe

them. If you don't feel much, that's okay too. There is no right or wrong way to have a body.

4 *Move up your body*: Slowly move your attention up through your body, taking time to notice sensations in each area:
  o Ankles and calves
  o Knees and thighs
  o Hips and pelvis
  o Lower back and abdomen
  o Chest and upper back
  o Shoulders and arms
  o Hands and fingers
  o Neck and throat
  o Face, including the jaw, mouth, nose, eyes, and forehead.
  As you focus on each area, notice any bracing patterns or if you are holding any tension. If you find tension, see if you can gently release it with each exhale.

5 *Acknowledge emotions and thoughts*: If any emotions or thoughts arise during the scan, acknowledge them without judgment. It's okay to feel whatever comes up. Just notice these feelings and thoughts. It may help to name them and gently bring your focus back to the body area you're scanning. For example, if you notice you are worried about something in your future, you might simply note "worry" or "future." More about repairing your nervous system in Chapter 8.

6 *End the scan*: Once you've scanned your entire body, take a moment to notice how your body feels as a whole. Take a few deep, grounding breaths. When ready, gently wiggle your fingers and toes, stretch if that feels good, and slowly open your eyes or lift your gaze.

7 *Reflection*: Take a moment to reflect on your experience. How does your body feel now compared to before the scan? Did you notice areas of bracing or holding tension in your body? You may find it helpful to journal about your experience. Note: *This step is optional.*

Please be patient with yourself. Some days, you might feel more connected to your body than others, and that's normal. Make this practice as long or short as you would like. You might find a quick version of this practice is more accessible throughout your day. It's okay to focus on just a few areas of your body where you typically feel tightness.

Slowing down lets your body know you are safe. Body scans calm the nervous system, promote relaxation, and improve overall body awareness. This practice can be particularly beneficial when you are experiencing anxiety, stress, or physical discomfort. I also recommend body scans to improve your sleep.

Journal prompts

Journaling can be a powerful tool for getting to know your nervous system and your patterns of dysregulation. Get to know your nervous system by using the prompts for a period of time, a few days to a week. Here are some prompts that may help you explore this:

1 *Physical sensations*: Describe any physical sensations you experienced today that got your attention. Did you feel tension, restlessness, or numbness? Where in your body did you notice these sensations?

2 *Emotional state*: What emotions did you experience today that were particularly interesting to you? Were there moments when you felt overwhelmed, anxious, or detached? How did these feelings manifest physically and mentally? For example, many people feel "butterflies in their stomach" when they are a little anxious or excited.

3 *Triggers*: Identify specific events or situations that triggered strong emotional or physical responses today or in your memory. What were they, and how did you react?

Note: *You can pass! Please take good care of yourself.*

4   *Behavioral responses*: Reflect on any behaviors you engaged in today that indicate that your nervous system was dysregulated (e.g., avoiding certain situations, distracting yourself with social media, or withdrawing). What was happening around you when these behaviors occurred?

5   *Thought patterns*: Do you have any habitual thought patterns that show up when you are distressed? For example, do you worry more about your eating, exercise, getting older, body size and shape, and health concerns? Are there recurring negative or anxious thoughts? How did these thoughts influence your actions and feelings?

6   *Coping mechanisms*: What strategies did you use to cope with stress or discomfort today? Were these strategies helpful or unhelpful? How did they impact your body's sensations or state of mind?

7   *Energy levels*: How was your energy level throughout the day? Did you experience fatigue, bursts of energy, or fluctuating energy levels?

8   *Social interactions*: How did your interactions with others go today? Did you feel more withdrawn, irritable, or overly engaged? How did your nervous system's state of regulation influence these interactions?

9   *Mindfulness and awareness*: Did you practice any mindfulness or grounding techniques today? If so, what were they, and how did they affect your awareness of your body's sensations and emotional well-being?

10 *Patterns and insights*: Looking back over the past week or month, identify any patterns in your physical sensations, emotional states, or behaviors that might indicate nervous system dysregulation. Do you have any insights into these patterns?

These prompts can help you gain a deeper understanding of how your nervous system responds to various experiences and practices. Another important area to consider is how your relationship with your body may relate to your nervous system.

Shame is a human experience

Shame is embarrassment or humiliation that arises from the perception that we have done something wrong, are flawed, and are no longer worthy of belonging or love. Guilt and shame are related, but guilt is feeling like we have done something bad, and shame is feeling like we *are* bad.

Experiencing shame regularly, without having a safe refuge or mending the damage of the experiences, leaves you feeling unworthy. Without conscious effort on your part, shame can even move from an experience to part of your identity. But it doesn't have to.

You can practice noticing your cues of dysregulation, so this does not happen. Think back to the list of common signs. Which ones have you felt when you have experienced shame? These are all signs that you need a safe refuge. Once you recognize this need, you can begin to reframe your thoughts, give yourself some kindness, and move through a shaming experience rather than dropping anchor and identifying with it. These are not easy changes but very possible shifts in how you talk and relate to yourself.

You need counterbalances, ideally acceptance from your relationships with others and, most importantly, in your relationship with yourself. These prevent shame from taking root. Co-regulating your nervous system with another person may require asking for what you need, which is also a practice. Sometimes, calling a friend or letting your family know you need a hug or a snuggle is precisely what your nervous system needs. Let's consider how the experience of shame relates to our shame about our bodies.

Body shame

Body shame is shame we experience related to our bodies. It stems from societal standards, media portrayals, peer and family values, and health and wellness industries. They all tell us and sell us the idea that certain body types—and the people that inhabit them—are more worthy than others.

Sally's story

Sally, a client in her late 40s, described a childhood experience of body shame that started her lifelong struggle with negative body image and disordered eating. When Sally was nine years old, she went to her friend's birthday party, a pool party. Someone took a photograph of her arm-in-arm with her besties, smiling wide, hair wet, wearing their swimsuits. This was back when photographs were sent away to be developed at a lab, so Sally forgot all about having her photo taken at the party.

When she saw the picture weeks later, body shame *washed* over her. Nine-year-old Sally hopelessly fixated on her belly, and she couldn't help comparing herself with her friends, with their flat stomachs. This photo, and the body shame it caused, set off a lifelong effort to change her body's size and shape. Specifically, changing her belly.

Sally actually brought the photograph into her session to share along with her story. She had kept it, all these thirty-odd years later. Of course, when she shared the photograph wt me I saw a "normal" nine-year-old girl who looked very happy with her friends.

As we talked about this memory and her childhood more generally, she realized that, growing up, her family highly valued health and fitness. Her body was never a topic of conversation, but she often heard her parents judge the bodies of others. Being an intuitive and sensitive child, she internalized the message that some bodies were good and some were not. She associated her nine-year-old belly with the bodies she often heard her parents judge as "bad." The body shame Sally experienced became embedded in her identity, preoccupying, and altering her relationship with her body from that moment forward.

But body shame does not only come from experiences with our families; it may result from one-off encounters and systems baked into our culture, such as:

- *Your lived experience*: Negative experiences such as bullying, teasing, or rejection based on appearance understandably lead to feeling body shame.

- *Internal criticism*: Most of us internalize messages, stories, and beliefs about our bodies, which develop during harmful experiences and due to societal or peer pressure. These experiences commonly lead to internalized body criticism and dissatisfaction unless these negative stories are challenged and dismantled.

- *Social contagion*: When friends, family, or peers make comments or jokes about your, their, or another's appearance, this intentionally or unintentionally contributes to your feelings of body shame.

- *Culture's health/beauty ideals*: Our culture promotes a narrow health and beauty ideal through media, advertising, pop culture, influencers, celebrities, and the medical industrial complex. These standards can make you feel that your body is not enough, too much, flawed, and inadequate.

- *Distortions by technology*: Constant exposure to edited and filtered unrealistic images of "ideal" bodies alongside a significant lack of body diversity can create a distorted perception of what is "normal" or worthy.

- *Cultural factors*: What happens when the bodies of your ancestors, lineage, family, or cultural identity are rarely represented? What happens when the dominant image of health and beauty ideals does not reflect your heritage or identity? Seldom, if ever, seeing a body like yours represented in the media can affect how you feel about your body, making it much more challenging to see your body as worthy or enough.

As Tressie McMillan Cottom says in her book *Thick: And Other Essays*, "Beauty isn't actually what you look like; beauty is the preferences that reproduce the existing social order."

Body break

Body shame and critical body stories are likely dysregulating to you, so please take a moment to take care of yourself. These are also opportunities to heal your relationship with your body. Here is a simple body, or somatic, practice if you want to try it.

Begin by making yourself as comfortable as possible. Feel your feet or your seat, and scan your body for places you may be bracing or holding patterns of tension. Focus on them and release and soften. Inhale your shoulders to your ears and exhale with a sigh as you let them drop. Do that as many times as feels good to you. Breathe.

If you can offer one statement of kindness to your body, speak this to yourself as you inhale. Speaking to your body this way may initially feel false or just plain weird. That's okay. Try it again.

Return to this practice several times in the next few minutes and then again later in your day and over the coming week. Over time, you may experience an opening to authentic kindness for your amazing aging body.

Before we get into some challenging truths about how hard it is to have a body, especially in this culture, please take good care of yourself if this has stirred up some dysregulation. Try another body practice or take a break before continuing. You are not alone. Remember that you are safe in this moment. We are all in this healing process together.

Body hierarchy

I've mentioned the body hierarchy earlier, but this topic is of such great importance that I want to make sure you understand its relevance to your relationship with your body and body shame. Let's dig into it a little more deeply now.

Back to Sally's story of body shame. I can't help but wonder how she would have felt about seeing her body reflected in the photograph if she had not internalized her parents' body judgments and values. How would she have reacted if the world around her valued all bodies equally, where she had not learned that there was a right and a wrong way to have a body? Or what if she lived in a culture that celebrated body diversity? Of course, we'll never know because such a thing was rare in our childhood, lifetimes, or current experiences.

We live in a world with a very real body hierarchy. In our current Western colonized construct, the top of that ladder is:

- White
- Thin
- Young
- Able-bodied
- Cis-gender
- Heterosexual
- Masculine.

And so, those who hold these identities have a sense of belonging and even power without earning that place. In her must-read book, *The Body Is Not an Apology*, Sonya Renee Taylor calls these the "default" bodies, the bodies we think about when we think of humans. Those with "other than" these identities are pushed to the margins and feel the need to earn their way into belonging and, therefore, safety. All the systems that make you feel "greater than" someone or "less than" someone are part of the ladder of the body hierarchy.

If this is a new concept for you, or if you doubt the validity of a body hierarchy in our culture, think about it this way. You may relate to the experience of joining a group of people or attending an event and scanning the room to see how your body size, age, gender, skin tone, etc., compares to the others. In minutes, you know how you "stack up." Your comparison based on the body hierarchy gives you a sense of "where you stand." And if you find others who share your identity, you feel more secure, less alone or threatened.

This body hierarchy has been a part of your experience for so long that you are likely unaware of it. But it is a very real part of our human experience. We live in a culture with systems that uphold the body hierarchy. Are these systems affecting your relationship with your body?

Your body in systems of oppression

Let's start with your family system. What did you learn from your parents or caregivers that blocked feeling comfortable and confident in your body? Is there one incident or a series of incidents, like in Sally's home, that reinforced the idea of right and wrong bodies?

How about your experience in the educational system? What did you learn about eating and exercise or your body's worth in school?

What about the marital or dating relationship system? Do you feel lovable just as you are? I sure hope so, but I know it's sadly not the case for everyone.

How about the healthcare system and the diet/wellness culture embedded in it? What did your interactions with doctors, nurses, and even medical receptionists tell you—explicitly or implicitly—about your body and how you care for it? Based on the stories I've heard from hundreds of clients, I'm sure you learned more ideas than you can count that made you feel less worth about your body while seeking healthcare.

How about our economic system or capitalism? How do you think capitalism benefits from you doubting that you are okay the way you are?

Even the religious system you are a part of may have contributed to how you feel about your body. Sadly, many of my clients learned more about dieting and the value of thinness at their place of worship. This experience comes to life in *The Way Down: God, Greed, and the Cult of Gwen Shamblin*, a docuseries examining the rise of the controversial Remnant Fellowship, a weight loss-based Christian church, and its late founder.

If you feel like ageism and diet culture are everywhere, you are quite right. It is everywhere. Body hierarchy permeates Western society—even in what we may consider our safest places.

We believe we will be safe, secure, worthy, and good enough if our bodies appear closer to the default body. We believe we will continue to belong, have social collateral, or remain relevant if we look fit, youthful, and hip. The pressure from so many of our social systems grinds us down and diminishes our comfort with our bodies, making us excellent anti-aging/longevity and diet/wellness culture consumers.

The lie of diet/wellness culture

Diet culture would have you believe that you have mastery over your body size and shape by controlling your food intake and exercise. *That is a lie.*

Research resoundingly supports that it's not all down to your individual choices, the way diet culture wants you to believe. Even if everyone ate the same diet and moved exactly the same, we'd still have bodies of varying sizes, shapes, and compositions. Your body's size, shape, and composition are influenced by:

- Genetics
- Life experiences and circumstances
- Your access to healthcare, food and safe spaces for movement
- Disease processes
- Injuries
- Age
- Medications
- The diets and experiences of your ancestors (epigenetics).

Bodies come in all shapes and sizes, and there is no wrong or right way to have a body. Body judgment is based on a social construct, the body hierarchy, which is passed down from generation to generation.

You may be thinking, "But what about health?" Diet culture promotes the belief that we are concerned about larger bodies because weighing more "causes" poor health outcomes. This belief is oversimplified and based on flawed thinking.

For a deeper dive into this topic, I have included excellent resources at the end of the book. Educating yourself about the lies of diet culture and anti-fat bias is likely to bring fascination, rage, and heartbreak. When my clients first wake up to the lies of diet culture and learn about how anti-fat bias has affected their medical care and other aspects of their lives, it takes time to process the mash-up of thoughts and feelings. The beautiful part of this process is that there is also a new capacity for self-compassion and empowerment.

Healthism

For most of us, "healthy" means being free of illness and feeling well. However, when "healthy" describes a behavior or food choice, we enter morality territory. Does making a healthy choice mean you are being "good"?

The sociologist Robert Crawford coined the term "healthism" in the 1980s. Healthism describes a societal trend where health and wellness are overly prioritized and moralized, often to the extent that your worth and value are judged based on your health status and lifestyle choices.

Let's explore healthism in more depth and consider how it might affect our relationship with our bodies. Healthism shows up as:

- *Moralization of health*: Health is seen as a moral imperative, where being healthy is equated with being virtuous and responsible. People who maintain healthy lifestyles are often viewed as disciplined and morally superior, while those who do not are considered lazy or irresponsible.

- *Individual responsibility*: You are personally responsible for your health, ignoring broader social, economic, and environmental factors that impact your well-being. Complex health issues are boiled down to your individual choices alone. You are encouraged to adopt health-promoting behaviors (e.g., diet, exercise) and are often blamed if you experience health issues.

- *Medicalization of daily life*: Everyday behaviors and choices are scrutinized through a medical lens, focusing on preventing disease and optimizing health. Your ordinary life experiences (e.g., aging, stress) are pathologized and treated as medical issues to be managed. Healthism blames you for your health conditions without considering external influences and the more complex experience of aging.

- *Commercialization and consumerism*: The wellness industry capitalizes on healthism by promoting products and services that falsely promise better health, commonly without scientific data. Yet, these products and services are entirely unregulated. Despite this, you are encouraged to spend money on fitness programs, supplements, health foods, and other wellness products.

- *Social inequality*: Healthism exacerbates social inequalities by privileging those with the resources and access to maintain a healthy lifestyle. Those from lower socioeconomic backgrounds face stigma and discrimination if they are unable to meet the societal standards of health. Healthism stigmatizes those who are ill or have disabilities, reinforcing ageism, ableism, and weight stigma.

- *Impact on mental health*: The pressure to achieve and maintain an ideal state of health can lead to anxiety, stress, and other mental health issues. This can turn obsessive, leading to disordered eating, excessive exercise, and other harmful behaviors.

Understanding healthism is essential for a more balanced and inclusive approach to your health that recognizes the internalized cultural factors that may be contributing to your well-being.

As you age, do you feel like prioritizing your health is your moral imperative? Or your choice? Do you feel pressured to "work" to stay healthy and stigmatized if you are not hopping on the "healthy" bandwagon? These theoretical questions relate to our conversation about your nervous system. You feel safe if you join in on what our culture deems as a priority and a worthy way to live your life. If you make a different choice, you may feel alone and even stigmatized, which your nervous system experiences as a threat, making you vulnerable to dysregulation. I'm sure you can remember how being "the odd one out" feels.

Hear me out. I am not saying that prioritizing health is wrong or a problem. What you do to support your health and well-being is your personal choice. Rather, I want to help you understand how healthism contributes to ageism, ableism, and anti-fat bias, which influence your relationship with your body and contribute to your nervous system dysregulation.

You cannot tell by looking at someone's body size, shape, or age that they are healthy.

I know that's a bold statement! You can be fat and metabolically well and even fit. I once worked with a client who could not buy clothing in most stores and whose personal trainer told me she was the most fit client he had ever worked with. You can also certainly be a thin person and metabolically unwell and unfit. Diet culture reduces our perception of a person's well-being and even worth to their size and appearance.

Saying that being fat "causes" disease is not precisely true. There are several confounding factors to consider:

- Weight cycling, or yo-yo dieting, is an independent health risk. Most people who are fat have been on multiple diets and have experienced weight cycling, so how can you separate a person's risk factor for being fat vs. weight cycling?
- Experiencing weight stigma causes a physiological stress response. Chronically experiencing stress is a well-documented health risk. So, weight stigma (rather than actual body weight) is another independent health risk.
- Healthcare providers may hold biased attitudes toward patients with higher body weight, leading to inadequate care, misdiagnoses, or delayed treatment.
- Patients may avoid seeking medical help due to fear of being judged or shamed for their weight.
- Weight stigma can also contribute to disordered and damaging eating behaviors.
- Weight stigma can also contribute to avoidance of physical activity due to fear of judgment.

Yes, there is a correlation, but we do not have evidence of causation. We do, however, have evidence of weight stigma in healthcare and all other aspects of our culture.

Let's dig deeper into weight stigma and why it may contribute to the dysregulation of your nervous system.

Weight stigma

Weight stigma refers to the discrimination, stereotyping, and prejudice directed at individuals based on their body weight, especially those with higher body weights. This stigma is real and pervasive in all areas of society, including healthcare, education, employment, media, fashion, and personal relationships. Remember the body hierarchy: bodies that do not appear thin are pushed to the margins.

Weight stigma is a health risk. Numerous studies have shown that exposure to weight stigma changes your stress responses in a way that indicates chronic stress, just like exposure to racism and other forms of systemic oppression.

What we internalize is the most complex and harmful weight stigma. Diet culture teaches you that your body is a problem. Since dieting typically does not lead to weight loss over time, you begin to lose trust in yourself and doubt your worth.

Diet culture, weight stigma, and anti-fat bias are aspects of the most pervasive systemic oppression of all-white supremacy and patriarchy.

White supremacy, patriarchy, and diet culture

"… the current anti-fat bias in the United States and much of the West was not born in the medical field. Racial scientific literature since at least the eighteenth century has claimed that fatness was 'savage' and 'black.'"

Dr. Sabrina Strings, Fearing the Black Body:
The Racial Origins of Fat Phobia

At this point, I hope you are starting to see the pervasive prevalence of diet culture and weight stigma. We are bombarded with these messages all the time and once you start to notice it, it feels like it's everywhere and all the time. Not only is toxic diet culture a harmful influence on your feelings of worth, body image, eating, movement, and your relationship with your body and food—it also has its roots in white supremacy that lives on today as an oppressive system in our lives. If this is something you've never considered, it helps to learn more about why we see some bodies as superior or inferior to others. No shade to anyone here! We've simply been swimming in these waters, not recognizing that we are even in water.

Diet culture is directly related to anti-fat bias because diet culture values thinness over everything else. Dr. Strings creates a compelling case for the historical roots of anti-fat bias in how bodies were judged during the trans-Atlantic slave trade. White European colonists labeled Black bodies as gluttonous, undisciplined, and hypersexual and held that their love of food made them fat. Meanwhile, the European and Puritan colonizers considered themselves superior due to their "self-control and moderation," which they believed were responsible for thinness.

In addition to imposing European beauty standards on enslaved and indigenous peoples, during the late 19th and early 20th centuries, scientific racism and eugenics promoted certain body types, particularly those of white Europeans, as inherently superior. These pseudoscientific beliefs reinforced the desirability of thinness as a marker of racial superiority.

Media in predominantly white societies has historically prioritized and amplified thin, young, non-disabled white women as the epitome of beauty. This representation pushes diverse bodies (older, larger, disabled, Black, Indigenous, People of Color) or outside this exclusionary standard of beauty to the margins. I am living in a white, straight-sized body, so I interviewed someone who can speak from her lived experience.

Notes from an expert

Sawanda Spinks is a mental health practitioner, mindset and confidence coach, and author of *Weightless Wisdom: How to Break Free from Diet Culture and Embrace Your NOW Body*:

We know that you can stay psychologically enslaved by diet culture. Generations have been lied to, and told that we were not good enough. I was told that I was not good enough because of my weight, because of what I eat, because of how I eat. The messages I received were, "Oh, no, you gotta do better. And here's how you have to do better. You have to conform." And I tried to do that for decades, since I was 12 years old.

I was called "fat," but it was "fat, black, ni**er." That's what I heard, all at one time, and it stung because I'd never heard the third word before. I'd never heard that until a white boy called me that. In middle school I was at a private school with

> very few black children. And I was bigger than everybody. With that came ridicule. And so it was like, well, maybe I do need to conform, you know. I wanted to fit in.

Patriarchy also enforces strict beauty standards on women, valuing them primarily for their appearance and conformity to these standards. Diet culture exploits this by promoting the idea that a woman's worth is tied to her ability to achieve and maintain a specific body type or appearance. This reinforces gendered power dynamics, where women are pressured to conform to male-defined ideals of beauty.

> "Diet culture encourages constant monitoring and control of one's body with rigid control over eating and movement, perpetuating the idea that bodies, especially women's bodies, must be controlled and disciplined. This is a form of social control that aligns with patriarchal regulation of women's autonomy and freedom. "A culture fixated on female thinness is not an obsession about female beauty, but an obsession about female obedience. Dieting is the most potent political sedative in women's history; a quietly mad population is a tractable one."
>
> *Naomi Wolf, The Beauty Myth*

White supremacy and patriarchy are intertwined with and show up as diet culture through the historical impositions of Eurocentric beauty standards, gender norms, and psychological impacts. We have to recognize these connections to deconstruct these harmful ideals and promote a more inclusive and equitable understanding of beauty and health on a macro and micro level. My clients find it very helpful to recognize and understand these long-standing cultural standards and how they affect how they experience their bodies. I hope this helps you dismantle these internalized beliefs that you limit your ability to nourish and care for your body without the old idea that your body is wrong and needs to be fixed. And what about the additional layer of ageism?

Ageism—another layer of oppression

Ageism intersects with other forms of oppression, such as anti-fat bias, sexism, racism, and ableism, compounding the effects of being marginalized. Ageism and diet culture are related primarily through their shared emphasis on unrealistic and often harmful societal standards, particularly around appearance and healthism. Ageism involves negative stereotypes about aging, promoting the idea that as we grow older, we should look and act a particular way to be considered attractive or valuable.

The combined pressures from the beauty, diet, and wellness industries capitalize on both ageism and anti-fat bias, marketing products and services that promise to reverse signs of aging or achieve a particular body size and shape. This perpetuates the idea that aging is undesirable and that we should continually strive to look younger in addition to looking thinner. This pressure is so commonplace that you may not even recognize how exhausting it is to feel you must constantly work on your body!

The pressure from both ageism and diet culture can lead to adverse psychological effects, such as:

- Poor body image
- Disordered eating
- Anxiety
- Depression
- Low self-esteem.

Growing older may have you considering a more extreme diet or exercise regimen to meet societal expectations. Ageism and diet culture both marginalize humans who do not fit the "default" criteria, which is isolating and dysregulating. But you don't have to believe these cultural stories or succumb to sociocultural pressures! These beliefs are learned and can be unlearned and dismantled. You can break free from these constraints.

Where body shame and dysregulation meet

All of these society-wide systems, diet/wellness culture, healthism, weight stigma, white supremacy, patriarchy, ageism, and more contribute to your individual moments of body shame.

You've likely had an experience that triggered body shame, and the shame that "washed over you" or "flew all over you" when you heard a triggering comment around you or you saw something triggering. This body sensation is your nervous system on body shame. Body shame can negatively impact your feelings of worth, leading to serious consequences if left unchecked.

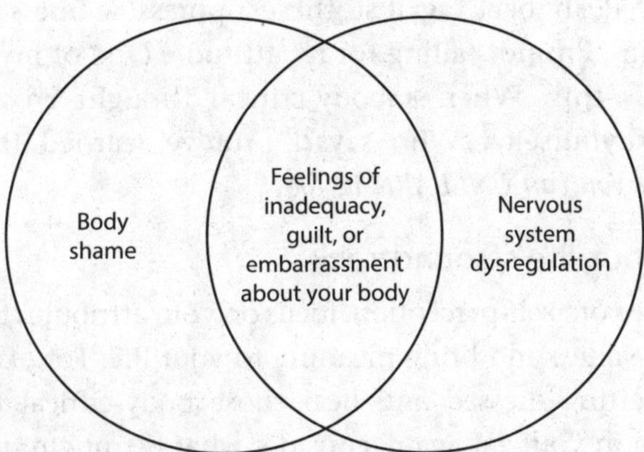

Body shame lingers and leads to feelings of inadequacy, guilt, or embarrassment about your body or appearance and contributes to anxiety, depression, disordered eating, body dysmorphia, and other issues. If these negative feelings about your body persist, they lower your overall feelings of worth and confidence. As a result, you may limit yourself by avoiding putting yourself out there and saying "Yes" to life or avoiding social situations, activities, or intimacy to protect yourself from potential judgment and embarrassment. Body shame may also be a chronic stressor in your life, negatively impacting your physical health. Commonly, it can also lead to disordered relationships with your eating and exercise.

Mending your body shame

I am thrilled that picking up this book is a part of mending your body shame! Here are some of my favorite suggestions gleaned from my many years of working with clients who are working to heal body shame (along with mending my body shame).

Media literacy

Start by educating yourself about the unrealistic nature of the bodies portrayed in the media that are heavily curated and digitally altered to meet narrow beauty/health ideals and standards. Push back against these oppressive messages and embrace an "I'm not falling for it" attitude. One of my favorite practices is this: When a body-critical thought crosses your mind, ask yourself, "Who says?!" You've learned this body judgment. *You can UNLEARN it, too.*

Create your life's soundtrack

To improve your self-perception, focus on your attributes that align with your values and bring meaning to your life. For example, if you are getting dressed and hear those body-critical thoughts whispering in your ear again, consider what is truly important to you and how your body supports you in doing just that. Or think of those you love and ask if their bodies are significant to you. Most of us think of how our loved ones make us feel, their sense of humor, kindness, courage, and many other things.

Remember, your body is your life partner, not your life's project.

The process of mending your body shame is more than a one-and-done endeavor. You will likely need to practice these shifts and reframes frequently to experience a change in your body shame. The work of healing this body shame is challenging but worthwhile, freeing up so much space in your head and heart.

Cultivate your support

Surrounding yourself with supportive and nonjudgmental people goes a long way! You may also realize that you need to set some boundaries.

Protect yourself with boundaries

Mending your body shame will mean growing fresh perspectives and new skills. This new growth is likely vulnerable at first. You know what I mean if you are a gardener or a lover of house plants. New growth on a plant is the most vulnerable area and should be protected from harsh and toxic elements. The same goes for you as you mend your relationship with your body. Protect yourself from harmful sources of body criticism; unfollow or mute accounts, change your media consumption habits, and even have an awkward conversation or two with some people in your life.

Promote diversity

Curating the media you consume by encouraging and embracing diverse body types normalizes that bodies come in all shapes, sizes, ages, colors, abilities, and gender identities. Expanding the images of bodies you are exposed to helps you expand your definition of beauty and health! See the Resources section for supportive media with images that are sexy, beautiful, joyful, vital, expressive—and diverse!

Self-compassion

Practices like mindfulness and self-compassion can help you begin to accept and respect, maybe even appreciate, your body. I've included a body-compassion practice in Chapter 7.

So, while it is of great importance that we identify and heal our body shame, it is of little ultimate good if we do not address the systems in which we learn our body shame.

Mending your body shame around aging with aging body liberation

Addressing ageism and diet culture requires challenging these societal standards, promoting diverse representations of beauty and health, and fostering a more inclusive understanding of aging and body diversity. There are just as many ways to have a body as there are to live your life and grow older.

Remember the body hierarchy we talked about earlier? You have likely internalized it unless you've started to recognize and challenge the sociocultural beliefs you've inherited. We must dismantle our internalized body hierarchy to be free of these confining definitions of beauty, health, and aging.

To destroy this hierarchy inside yourself, you must ask yourself some hard questions to divest from these oppressive systems:

- Where does the system live inside of me?
- Am I comparing myself to others? Can I notice this habit and confront these patterns?
- How am I judging myself and my body based on this hierarchy?

Our desire for proximity to the default body breathes life into the hierarchy. It's understandable to want to hold onto a sense of belonging, to feel relevant and powerful. This is not about judging yourself for judging yourself! This is about becoming aware of these habitual patterns both inside and outside you so that you can become curious about how this affects you and, specifically, your relationship with your body. These habitual patterns keep the body hierarchy alive. As with most changes in the world, this starts with you. When you begin to see that you've bought into this, you recognize in yourself:

- I've bought into wanting thinness.
- I've bought into wanting to look younger.
- I've bought into desiring to be able-bodied and independent.
- Have I explored my relationship to LGBTQIA+ bodies, queerphobia, or transphobia?
- Have I explored my relationship with racism?
- Have I explored my relationship with ageism and ableism?
- Have I explored my relationship with sexism?

You live within multiple systems that affect how you see bodies, including your own. These systems uphold the body hierarchy. The goal is to ask yourself these questions, and the hierarchy will weaken and fall, starting with your internalized body hierarchy.

With this new lens, you can liberate yourself from the limiting beliefs and systems of oppression. Then, you get to decide how you want to create your next chapter and how you want to age.

Now, let's get this party started! I'm so excited about Part 2, where we'll discuss principles and practices for mending your relationship with your body and how you care for yourself with nourishment, movement, rest, and nervous system regulation. Let's go!

2
MENDING

Your body is your life partner

5

Nourishing your body respect

I'm exhaling—and I hope you are too!—now that we've arrived at Part 2! This part pivots away from all of the ways ageist diet/ wellness culture has damaged your relationship with your body and socialized you to believe your body is not enough, too much, and a project that you need to be working on relentlessly. In this section, we dismantle those beliefs and mend that fractured relationship through how you eat, move, rest, and overall relate to your body. This chapter focuses on nourishing your relationship with your body, while breaking free from ageism and diet/wellness culture constraints.

This chapter asks you to look away from the seductive side of what restrictions and following food rules may have promised, cultivate the capacity to look inward with respect for your body's wisdom and develop a relationship with your body as your partner. You'll focus on eating enough by honoring your body's hunger and practicing flexibility with your eating choices based on what is accessible, satisfies, and sustains you. This chapter also weaves in new concepts to reclaim a healthy body partnership by attending to, passionately listening, asking for consent, and building trust with your body.

I grew up in a small town in North Carolina, and my grandmother lived next door. Her backyard garden, apple trees, grapevine, magical chicken and dumplings, and famous pound cake filled my belly and childhood with love and wonder. It's funny what sticks with you: the smell of warm biscuits and the way she whipped honey and butter together, taking her simple biscuits to another level; her heavy hand with the pepper shaker as she prepared scrambled eggs for me when I slept over (a preference that remains with me); the large tin salt shaker that she kept on the picnic table on the back porch for the specific purpose of salting watermelon in the summer. I have many delicious memories of time spent by her side in her kitchen. My expansive interpretation of what it means to be nourished is rooted in these childhood experiences. I realize now that one of my true privileges is that food was never reduced to its nutritional value in my childhood. I've wondered many times how this might have protected me.

"To nourish" means "to provide the food or other substances necessary for growth, energy, and health." The word "nourish" comes from the Latin verb *nūtrīre*, meaning "to feed" or "to care for." Yes, and so much more. This chapter shows you a more expansive view of nutrition than you'll find in popular culture. We'll add the essential elements of pleasure and satisfaction to how nutrition is typically discussed—**nutrition + pleasure/ satisfaction = nourishment.**

The pivot—turning away from diet/wellness culture rules

When my clients successfully break free from following external food rules, and spending time in their heads counting, calculating, and tabulating what they are eating, I hear comments like:

- "I'm noticing that I'm not beating myself up about my eating the way I used to."
- "I feel more connected to my body in ways I don't think I have since I was a kid. I am in the same body, but I feel lighter and more at ease. Sometimes, I even feel confident."
- "I am not worrying about what I ate before I go to sleep and what I 'should' eat when I wake up. All of the space that used to be taken up by food obsessions is now free for other things!"

- "I am starting to notice how certain foods make me feel when I am not focused on controlling my weight. Like, I don't sleep well and wake up with indigestion when I eat late. Who knew?!"
- "When I eat out or order takeout, I don't spend forever fighting myself about making the 'right' choice. It feels more like getting to know what would satisfy and sustain me than a test of my willpower."
- "Now, when I go on vacation, I don't feel like I have to eat all the special occasion foods because they are no longer forbidden in my daily life. I don't come home after a vacation feeling like I need to do 'damage control' and start another diet."
- "When I go grocery shopping, I am not full of dread and anxiety, buying the foods that are 'good' and feeling ashamed of myself when I buy the 'bad' foods. I don't spend forever agonizing over my choices."

Listening to your body takes intentionality, practice, time, and a great deal of patience. This new way of approaching eating takes time and effort. There will be good days and bad. This process is not linear or straightforward. For most of my clients, there are lapses and periods of wanting to return to old dieting habits. This shift toward following your internal guidance can be messy!

I'm not going to lie, following food rules is simpler and may feel easier, but as we've established, it is not sustainable and causes harm! Yes, there are clear boxes to check, and the human brain loves order and transparent rules to follow. So, if you've followed diets with food rules, you've developed a more black-and-white and all-or-nothing way of seeing food and eating. You are either on the wagon or falling off the wagon. You are either eating "good" foods or "bad" foods. You are either being good or being bad. There is very little gray, middle ground, or some of this and some of that.

The thing is, the middle place is where you will get to know yourself, discover your patterns and deeper insights, connect with your body's wisdom, and finally feel relief from soul-sucking, disembodied diet rules. This process of befriending and repairing your relationship with your body will slowly unfurl for you with time and practice.

It requires more energy to drop the old rules and turn toward your own body and instincts for guidance. It also requires courage because you are stepping away from what is known into the unknown. Uncertainty can be frightening and anxiety-provoking. It's like if you were ever afraid of the dark, you know what stepping into the dark is like. It's scary at first. Then, when you realize you are okay and your eyes adjust, you start to find your way.

Consider this: if you stay with the known and continue to do the same thing, you will continue to get the same results. Keeping up with food rules will cause you to cycle on and off, in and out of the food rules of the next fad, the next program, and the next promised silver bullet. These rules include longevity and anti-aging food rules! So why doesn't following food rules work for the majority of us?

Wired for pleasure and survival

Let's start with our bodies' hard wiring for survival. If you've been around a baby, you recognize that specific cry that communicates, "I'm hungry!" It can't be confused with anything else because of its sense of urgency. That is because hunger is a legitimate threat to survival and should be taken seriously. Then, the baby also communicates an apparent loss of interest when satiety is met.

This system works beautifully to regulate our body's energy balance. But at some point, our well-meaning caregivers interfered with our body's well-designed system communicating our appetite. Due to this interference, we learned to doubt, question, and disconnect from our bodies. This fracturing was likely part of your body story, as discussed earlier in Part 1. The interference sounds something like this:

- "You can have dessert when you finish what's on your plate."
- "Are you sure you really need seconds?"
- "If you eat your vegetables, you can have more potatoes."
- "Oh, please eat this, he made this just for you."
- "You don't want to have a weight problem like me. You don't need to eat the bread."

At some point, you began to follow these types of external rules about how you nourished yourself. However well-intended, they compounded disconnection from your body. The consequence is no longer trusting your body, but your body is still wired to protect you from the threat of hunger.

When your beautifully designed metabolism signals you're undernourished and that you need fuel, your body tries to protect you by sending obsessive thoughts about food and eating and ultimately lowering your metabolism to match your intake of calories. This latter strategy protects the energy stores in your warehouse adipose or (fat cells), so you'll have energy if you need it later. At the same time, your mind sends you cravings for the foods the "rules" say are off-limits or bad. It *wants* you to experience pleasure and eat satisfying foods. Seeking pleasure and your survival are inextricably linked. For these reasons, restrictive food rules and the resulting deprivation and hunger make these plans with food rules unsustainable for most of us.

Your not being able to follow food rules is not your fault. Diets don't work.

You don't have to take my word for it. A wealth of research demonstrates the harm of restriction, which is included in the Resources section.

To make it even more interesting, your body adapts to carry more weight during perimenopause and menopause to *protect* you. When the estrogen level produced by your ovaries tanks, your fat cells expand to produce more estrogen. This is good news for you because estrogen helps prevent bone breakdown along with a host of other menopause symptoms. More weight around your middle guards your vital organs. As Dr Margo Maine concluded beautifully, "Your body has tremendous knowledge that you need to respect. Honor your body's wisdom, and be grateful for all your body does for you each day."

What happens when humans are undernourished?

During World War II, we needed to feed people who had been starved. But we didn't have sufficient data on how to refeed people safely, so researchers ran The Minnesota Starvation Experiment. College-aged conscientious objectors during the war volunteered for this study. For three months, they were fed their usual amount of food. Then, for six months, they were fed half of their usual amount of food.

During this period of being undernourished, the men were obsessed with food. They collected photographs and recipes. These were college-aged men in the 1940s, way before our food network and foodies on social media, so this was very unusual behavior. They also exhibited marked levels of:

- Anxiety
- Depression
- Mood swings
- Irritability
- Problems with memory
- Difficulty with sleep and focus
- Fatigue
- Loss of interest in their usual activities, including sex.

These men felt very cold, so cold that they required an external source of warmth, such as the sun or a warm shower, to warm them up. Their metabolic rates dropped an average of 40 percent.

When the restrictions lifted, the men exhibited unusual eating habits. They were unable to stop eating, gulped food, and ate quickly. It took the men an average of five months to return to their previous eating habits. Still, some did not return to their baseline. Notably, most subjects no longer showed the psychological characteristics exhibited when undernourished. **The brain is the organ most affected by an undernourished body.**

Does this sound familiar to you? Likely, these college-aged men in the 1940s did not also experience guilt about their eating behaviors. They also likely have yet to return to restricting their food again. Now consider how many diets you have tried in your lifetime and how many times you experienced binge eating following periods of restriction. Your body was trying to protect you from past, present, and future deprivation and hunger.

Coming to terms with loss due to diet culture

Learning how restrictive food rules have affected you and coming to terms with the fact that diet culture has harmed you opens up a variety of responses. Most likely, the ultimate feeling is that of loss. Acknowledging the loss of your time, energy, money, and attention to diet culture opens up genuine grief.

As one of my clients put it, "I can't believe I've spent so much of my life chasing this idea that my body was wrong. I feel like I've mostly punished myself and missed out on so much living, postponing many things until I fixed my body."

We know that grief is complex. Grief is an umbrella that includes various other emotions and mental states experienced in waves, not linearly. The way each of us experiences loss and grief is unique. Once you see that you have lost part of your lifetime and resources to useless and harmful diet culture, you will likely have feelings to process. The phases below are considered aspects of grief, experienced in no particular order or sequence. Instead of stages, grief is more like waves of mixed emotions. You may experience a variety of feelings, including shock, anxiety, exhaustion, or guilt. You may also experience ups and downs, and go back and forth between stages.

However, you may experience only some of these.

Stage	Example
Denial	When I find the right plan, I will be "successful."
Bargaining	I will return to the (fill in the blank) diet, lose some weight, and then work on body liberation.
Depression	I'm just so sad that I lost so much of my time to diet culture. I put off doing so many things until I lost weight. There's no getting that lost time and opportunities back.
Anger	I cannot believe I fell for all of those promises and how much money they scammed from me!
Acceptance	Once I saw diet culture for what it was, I could let go and move on.

You may experience a mish-mash of feelings, including shock, anxiety, exhaustion, or guilt. Your particular way of grieving will likely include ups and downs, and go back and forth between stages.

The added layer of finding yourself midlife or older and coming to terms with what you've lost to diet culture is complicated. If you've spent your lifetime pursuing the promises of diet culture, you may have more to grieve.

I've included coming to terms here because you cannot skip this step. A wise therapist I once shared clients with often said, "It's just like when you're playing on the monkey bars. You can't move to the next rung until you let go of the one you're holding." I know it's not easy, but you need to process your losses to diet culture to be able to move on.

The good news is that you don't have to let diet culture get in your way for the rest of your precious life! Before we discuss what it means to move on from diet culture, let's take a break to check in.

Body break

Give yourself the gift of becoming comfortable in your body. First, check in and connect with your body with subtle movement. You could inhale your shoulders up to your ears and exhale them as they drop with several breath cycles. Or take a few minutes to stretch your arms up as you inhale and then exhale as you fold forward any amount. Or simply inhale some length into the back of your neck and then exhale as you drop your left ear to your left shoulder and feel the stretch in the right side of your neck for as long as that feels interesting to you, then follow the same sequence on the other side.

After you've connected again to being in your body, give yourself the gift of noticing how you feel as you scan your body from your toes, up your legs, into your pelvis, your belly and chest, your arms, hands, neck, face, and head. Are there any places that would feel better with softening or simply feeling the warmth of your touch? Give your body your own kindness, care, and attention.

Journal prompts

The losses experienced due to participating in diet culture can be complex and deeply personal, so journaling can be a powerful tool to help process these feelings. Here are some prompts designed to guide reflection and healing:

1 *Name your losses*: Name what you realize you lost due to participation in diet culture. How have these losses impacted your life?
2 *Acknowledge your feelings*: What emotions are you feeling right now? Anger, sadness, confusion? Let yourself freely express these emotions on the page.
3 *Coping with change*: How has this affected your daily life? Can you think of strategies that would help you cope?

4 *Finding meaning*: How do you make sense of this loss? What lessons have emerged from your experiences with diet culture?
5 *Support network*: Who are the people who could help you process these feelings? Do you need to seek support from new connections?
6 *Self-compassion*: Write about how you are taking care of yourself. How can you show yourself kindness and compassion as you acknowledge these losses and feel these emotions?
7 *Moving on*: How do you envision moving forward without diet culture? What fears do you have, and what hopes?
8 *Acceptance*: What does acceptance mean to you in the context of these losses? Are you at a place of acceptance, or is it still a process for you?

These prompts can help you explore many facets of your grief, process your emotions, and ultimately find a path toward acceptance and healing.

When you are ready, let's move on and mend the fractures created by diet culture.

Mending your relationship with your body

"and I said to my body, softly, 'I want to be your friend.'
It look a long breath and replied, "I have been
waiting my whole life for this.'"

Nayyirah Waheed

You are in a relationship with your body.

Let that sink in.

This relationship is likely complicated: a mix of dislike, distrust, and hopefully plenty of wonder and gratitude. Your body is truly miraculous and beautiful! Perimenopause and menopause may have you feeling your body has betrayed you or that you are at war with your body. Yes, things do go wrong sometimes. But most of the time, your body has been steadfast and gotten you through. And by the way, post-menopause is a more stable and comfortable place. It gets better!

Your relationship with your body is complicated if you've inherited harsh criticism of your body, comparing yourself to unattainable and ridiculous ideals. You may have pushed your body and ignored its whispers and shouts for rest, nourishment, and pleasure. You may even have punished your body at times.

Please forgive yourself as much as you can!

You simply tried to be "good" and do the right thing. You were trying to protect yourself from the judgment of our thin—and youth-obsessed—culture. You may have been following advice from your cousin, an influencer, or even a healthcare provider. Diet culture taught you to push through your hunger, ignore your body's requests for rest, and even ignore pain and keep going.

Have you heard the phrase often used in fitness culture: "Pain is the sound of weakness leaving your body"? Even the language we use to describe the information we receive from our bodies is judgmental. The dominant message in our culture is that "urges" and "cravings" are to be ignored and conquered, certainly not trusted!

You did not create this mess, but you can repair the damage.

If you have learned how to rebuild trust in a relationship after it has been broken, you can take a similar approach to restoring trust in your relationship with your body. The key components are:

- Connection/listening
- Curiosity rather than judgment
- Consent asking
- Compassion.

Let's examine how these components rebuild trust with your body, including examples of how they apply to nourishing, moving, and resting your body while creating practices that foster mending the fractures created by diet culture.

Connection and listening to your body

Most of my clients say they live completely unaware of themselves from the neck down, and I get it. Modern lifestyle can leave you feeling rushed, distracted, disconnected, and disembodied. Then diet/wellness and anti-aging/longevity industries require you to ignore or even fight what your body's nudges, desires, and calls for nourishment, rest, and pleasure. For example, if you start to feel hungry around four o'clock in the afternoon, you might think, "It will be time for dinner in a couple of hours. I'll just wait and eat then. Snacks are bad anyway." But you feel famished by the time you eat dinner, and your body feels threatened by the hunger level you are experiencing (remember the Starvation Experiment?), so you eat quickly and past the point of fullness. Your body is trying to protect you, ensuring you get plenty of nourishment in response to the experience of being underfed.

To prevent this disrespect to your body, you must listen to your body's communication of hunger, satisfaction, and fullness and be more connected to it to listen for and receive these cues. Just a reminder: the longer we live, the more varied our experiences—and our bodies—become. That means our connections to our bodies evolve, too. If tuning into your body feels confusing or out of reach right now, you're not alone. Stay with me—we'll explore the barriers and how to navigate them together.

Here are some ways to cultivate more connection and listening to your body.

Mindfulness of your body

Mindfulness of your body is a practice in which you bring your attention to bodily sensations, movements, and physical experiences in the present moment. This practice creates the potential for a deeper connection with your body and your present-moment experiences.

Here are some aspects of mindfulness of your body. Some may work for you, and some may not, so simply take what appeals and leave the rest.

Breath awareness

Notice your breath moving in and out of your body. Feel the rise and fall of your chest, the expansion and contraction of your abdomen, the sensation of air entering and leaving your nostrils. Simply notice how your body naturally breathes without trying to change anything. Remember, you can trust your body to breathe! Connection begins with the simple act of slowing down and noticing. It won't always feel easy or accessible—and that's okay. What matters is that you keep coming back to it.

Body scan

Bring your attention to different parts of your body, from head to toe, noticing sensations such as bracing, holding tension, warmth, coolness, or the feeling of air or clothing against your skin. The goal is to become aware of your body's sensations. There is no right or wrong way here. Simply notice.

Awareness of movement

Pay attention to your body's movements during daily activities such as walking, eating, and even sitting. This involves noticing how your body feels, for example the movement of your feet on the pavement or your hands on the steering wheel. Can you slow down and notice the taste of your food?

Mindfulness of the body increases your connection to and awareness of bodily sensations. It also cultivates your ability to receive information the body is trying to communicate, such as hunger and fullness. Mindfulness of the body is part of what is called *interoception*.

More broadly, interoception is the awareness of your body's internal state. It involves your ability to receive and interpret signals from within your body, such as hunger, thirst, need for sleep, pain, and even the fact that you may be holding your breath. This internal awareness affects how you experience emotions, regulate your body's functions, and maintain your body's internal balance.

One way to think about interoception is a mind–body connection. Developing a more sensitive sense of interoception can lead to a more accurate read of your body's current state and needs.

Interoception, sometimes called the "eighth sense," complements the traditional five senses. It plays a fundamental role in your awareness of your body's energy needs and balance or hunger and fullness. We'll revisit interoception in Chapter 6, when we discuss movement, and Chapter 7, when we discuss your nervous system.

Cues from your body that you are hungry, satisfied, and full are more complex and often challenging to interpret, especially after you've ignored your body's messages and got it in your head in order to follow rules about your food and eating. Let's break it down.

Hunger check-in and journal prompts

The way you experience hunger is unique to you. It is affected by a wide variety of factors, including:

- Genetics
- Metabolism
- Medications
- Mood
- Anxiety
- Amount and quality of sleep
- Health
- Age

- Diet history
- Eating Disorder history
- Trauma history
- Neurodiversity
- Conscious awareness.

There are different types of hunger. There are different levels of hunger. Hunger can be nuanced and complex.

Connect with your body. Take a few minutes to notice where you are making contact with your seat and your feet. If it is comfortable to notice your breath, please do so. When you feel more in touch with your body, ask yourself these questions:

- Am I hungry?
- What am I hungry for?
- How hungry am I?
- How do I know I am hungry?
- Do I notice a physical sensation associated with hunger?
- Where do I feel the sensation?
- How would I describe it?
- Are there emotions that arise when I feel hungry?
- Does noticing my hunger trigger a thought pattern, or do I tell myself any stories when I sense I am hungry?

Robin's story

Robin, a 46-year-old Black math professor at a prestigious university, was referred to me by her therapist, who wanted her to reconsider another diet after chronically dieting to lose weight most of her adult life. Robin was considering a liquid diet program at the local medical center, but, at the same time, she was "sick and tired" of dieting and didn't think she could put herself through another one. Overall, she felt extremely lost. She said "How could I be so successful in everything else but such a failure with my eating and my weight?"

Robin's story began with the loss of her mother when she was five years old. Her father forbade Robin from talking about her mother and married another woman within the following year. Her family removed every trace of her mother from her home. Robin told this story with no noticeable emotion and said several times that her step-mother treated her "fine."

In the 4th grade, Robin went through puberty. Other kids and her siblings teased her for having "large breasts." And because her family was very religious, her parents encouraged her to "cover up." Shamed about her body, Robin always left home in more conservative clothing. The next year, Robin was sexually assaulted by a friend's father. She was too embarrassed to tell anyone and did not begin to talk about it until recently in therapy.

When Robin was in the 6th grade, her stepmother took her to her pediatrician because she was concerned about Robin's weight. Robin started her first diet with strict controls and restrictions on her food intake. Meanwhile, her siblings could eat as they wished. Robin soon started sneaking food, which she continued to do when alone, both at school and home. She cycled on and off diets throughout her teenage years and college. Things got worse in graduate school when she started to feel caught in cycles of restriction followed by binge eating and then back again to restricting.

Further complicating Robin's relationship with her body, her father commonly made judgmental and critical comments about women's bodies. He found women with thinner bodies more attractive and successful, and made statements of disgust when he saw women in larger bodies. Whenever Robin heard these types of comments, she said, "I would get an odd knot in my stomach."

Robin impressed me as being very sensitive, kind, and intelligent. She came to our first session wearing a tailored suit and was very "put together." Over time, as we went deeper into her body story, the secrets came out.

Over the past 30-odd years, Robin kept many secrets: how much she missed her mother; how lonely she felt in her family; her sexual assault. But, most crucial to my work with Robin: she had been sneaking food and cycling between restricting and bingeing, a secret she kept from her family, friends, and even herself.

When we discussed ditching her dieting and instead trusting her body to lead her choices about eating, Robin said she felt "completely disconnected" from her body. We created some soft structure about her eating, encouraging her to eat every three to four hours. We also talked about how she could start to be more neutral about food, working to drop her labeling of foods (and herself) as "good" and "bad." Our goal was to be less restrictive to decrease her feelings of deprivation, judgment, and hunger.

To connect with her body and strengthen her interoception, we worked closely with Robin's therapist, encouraging practices that create mindfulness of her body sensations, including her hunger and fullness. Robin was open to these concepts because she never wanted to diet again and wanted to feel more embodied. She thought this would also help her feel "more alive," which was important to her at this stage of her life. She said she was excited to try this because she was "tired of feeling numb."

Barriers to the mind–body connection

There are real barriers to being able to connect with your body. I don't want you to feel like you are "broken" if you don't know when you are hungry or full. These barriers might include:

- *Chronic stress*: Chronic stress or anxiety can dull or distort interoceptive signals. When your body is constantly in a heightened state of arousal, you adapt and lose your sense of normalcy.
- *Trauma*: Trauma can lead to dissociation from bodily sensations as a protective means of coping. This can result in a disconnection from interoceptive signals, making it hard to recognize or trust internal cues.
- *Cultural norms*: Your family or friends may have discouraged you from expressing or attending to bodily needs. Expressing feelings may have been discouraged or even shamed. This experience may have taught you to suppress or ignore your body's needs, such as hunger or fullness.
- *Neurodiversity*: Being neurodiverse may alter your ability to interpret internal sensations by dulling, distorting, or amplifying the intensity of sensations, confusing your understanding of interoceptive signals. For example, if you have ADHD, you may not sense hunger cues while hyperfocusing, or eat when you are not hungry as a form of stimulation during periods of understimulation.

- *Eating disorders*: Eating disorders can affect interoception. Certainly, eating disorders cause a disconnection with your hunger and fullness.

- *Diet culture and modern lifestyle*: The fast pace of modern life and constant distractions can make it easy to ignore or overlook internal signals—your interoceptive awareness atrophies when you chronically ignore your body. Diet culture contributes to this further by creating rules you follow and, therefore, ignores your body's sensations of hunger and fullness.

- *Medications*: Some medications may alter bodily sensations or compromise your ability to interpret interoceptive signals. For example, GLP-1s disconnect you from your ability to sense hunger, and due to slowed gastric emptying, interpreting fullness becomes very confusing.

- *Physical health*: Some physical conditions can affect your body's ability to send or process interoceptive signals. For instance, neuropathy can dull sensations in parts of the body, leading to a decreased awareness of your internal state.

- *Gadgets*: People who rely heavily on external cues (like schedules, social cues, or technology) to guide their behavior may lose touch with their internal signals. For example, eating based on the clock rather than hunger signals can weaken interoceptive awareness related to appetite. Gadgets that tell you when it is time to get up and move interrupt your body's urge to get up and move around.

- *Sensory overload*: Environments with excessive external stimuli make it difficult to notice or interpret your internal bodily sensations. This can occur in noisy, busy, or chaotic settings. Some are more sensitive to this than others.

Let's return to Robin's story and look for barriers to her mind-body connection. First, Robin was living in a large Black woman's body. Per the body hierarchy, she was pushed to the margins of our culture due to how others saw her body. She experienced micro-aggressions based on her body size, her race, and her gender identity, which caused her to feel chronically unwelcome, unsafe, and stressed. Sometimes, she was aware of this, and sometimes, she was so desensitized to them that she didn't have conscious awareness.

She had also experienced traumas with the loss of her mother and the sexual assault. The suppression of her feelings related to her mother's death and the sexual assault and likely other needs as a child, along with the suppression of her hunger and fullness through her chronic dieting and the development of disordered eating, all contributed to a fracture of the mind-body connection and damaged her capacity for interoception.

The good news: Robin was highly motivated to mend her relationship with her body. She had a strong drive to feel embodied and vital again. Her commitment to working with her therapist, including somatic therapies, and working with me to incorporate practices that, with time, allowed her to notice her body's appetite, nourish herself, connect with, and trust her body again made her much more comfortable with her eating and body relationship.

But keep in mind, Robin had the privilege of access to care and the time and energy to devote to her healing. She also had a partner and a close friend who were very supportive of her recovery process.

In all, Robin felt some relief after the first six months. Due to the complications of trauma and how young she was when she started dieting, Robin's healing process took two to three years (depending on what level of healing we're talking about). Her level of motivation and readiness to ditch dieting and dive into her recovery made a significant impact on her progress.

You can improve your interoceptive awareness by integrating mindfulness practices, therapy (predominantly somatic and trauma-informed approaches), and intentional listening to your body's hunger and fullness cues. It may be helpful to track your hunger and fullness as you go through your day. I've provided a

Hunger and Fullness Scale with directions and more information about following your body's hunger and fullness cues.

These practices support you in learning to trust your body's cues and wisdom. Keep going!

Hunger and body respect

Turning away from following the "shoulds" and the rules you've learned about food and eating takes courage! You are swimming against the current of cultural anti-aging and diet culture norms, and you may feel lost and alone. That is precisely why I wrote this book, so I just want to congratulate you on making this brave choice. Getting to know your body's hunger, satisfaction, and fullness may be one of the most helpful parts of this process.

By ditching diet culture, you can turn inward and discover your body's cues. Start with a conversation with yourself about your hunger. When you begin to think about eating, check in with yourself and inquire, "Am I hungry?" Noticing your hunger *sounds* simple, but you may find that it isn't easy. However, this is an essential step in the process. It may take some time to begin to wake up your connection with your body and your body's cues.

Try experimenting with utilizing a Hunger–Fullness Scale. This concept was made famous by Evelyn Tribole and Elyse Resch's book *Intuitive Eating: A Revolutionary Anti-Diet Approach*. This scale will help you discover the nuances of your hunger, satisfaction, and fullness and strengthen your mind-body connection. Here is an example of one way to interpret the scale.

Hunger–Fullness Scale practice

Take a sheet of paper and draw a line down the middle, placing the number 1 at one end and the number 10 at the opposite end, very much like the one below, except you find your own description of how it feels to be empty at a 1, neutral at a 5, and extremely full at a 10. Track your hunger and fullness throughout the day for a few days. When you start thinking about food and eating, name your hunger level. When you are eating, name your fullness level. You may want to do this practice on and off every few weeks until you feel you've got the hang of it.

Rating	Description
0	Painfully hungry
1	Ravenous
2	Very hungry
3	Hungry
4	Mild hunger
5	Neutral
6	Mild fullness
7	Complete fullness
8	Slightly too full
9	Stuffed
10	Painfully full

Adapted from: "Hunger and Fullness Scale." *Nutrition and Food Services*, US Department of Veterans Affairs, July 2023, www.nutrition.va.gov/docs/ UpdatedPatientEd/HungerandFullnessScaleJul2023.pdf#.

Proceed with caution: If you are trying to ditch diet culture rules and jump into concepts of Intuitive Eating (IE) and the Hunger–Fullness scale, you may find that you approach this too with a diet culture mindset. You may think you must be hungry from your stomach, or physiologically hungry, to eat or give yourself permission to be "good" or doing IE "right." I encourage you to allow yourself to get messy with this process. Sometimes, you will eat because you are emotionally uncomfortable or emotionally "hungry," and that's okay. It is very human and normal to eat for emotional reasons. Please give yourself some compassion, and be curious about your experience.

The more you get to know yourself, the more you will recognize your patterns and begin to recognize and name your needs. With this discovery process, you have the opportunity to identify and meet your needs in various ways, including eating instead of only eating. For example, you may find that you:

- Eat when you are bored in the evenings
- Eat when you are antsy or dysregulated at the end of the day or when you are in a transition
- Eat to numb yourself or regulate your nervous system when you are feeling overwhelmed and dysregulated
- Eat when you were not satisfied by the food you ate earlier
- Eat to feel more full because that helps you feel more secure
- Eat when you feel emotionally depleted like your cup is empty
- Eat when you are tired
- Eat when you are happy and want to celebrate
- Eat as a way to connect with others
- And on it goes.

All of the above is normal! And once you know this about yourself, you can start making real changes. For instance, if you eat when you are bored in the evenings, you can pull out some of your art or crafting supplies instead or sign up for a class that regularly meets during this time. If you eat when you are antsy or dysregulated at the end of the day, you can practice yoga or use an app for guided meditations. Think of these gentle experiments to explore what supports your well-being. Lean into your curiosity rather than a "fix it" attitude.

Typically, we associate food with positive memories. Food and eating is a source of pleasure. Eating food lets our bodies know we are safe. Feeling fed often feels secure. So, eating is emotionally complex. My recommendations for you are to:

- Practice mindful awareness of your eating experiences and patterns. You will find a Mindful Eating Practice included in the Resources

- Offer yourself compassion when you feel like you are "messing up"
- Develop nonjudgmental curiosity about your eating
- Experiment with noticing and meeting your needs when you become aware of emotional eating patterns
- Remember it is normal and okay to eat for emotional reasons!

Pro-tips

- *Don't get too hungry*: One of the most essential strategies as you begin to nourish your body with respect is to try not to get too hungry. If you've experienced an eating disorder, chronic dieting, or food insecurity for any reason, your body has been under-fueled in the past. Your body feels threatened when you get too hungry and will send you urgent requests to eat past fullness to protect your body. This is why the restrict–binge cycle is so very common. You are unique, but most people *need to eat about every 3–4 hours to prevent getting too hungry.*

- *Carry food with you*: Carrying food with you when you leave home can provide you with more security and prevent you from getting too hungry. This is also a form of no longer neglecting yourself and prioritizing your body and nourishment in your life. *You deserve to be cared for and fed well.*

- *Eat satisfying foods*: If you are trying to depend on your body's cues for direction, such as when to eat, when to stop eating, and even what to eat, you must tune in to what is satisfying. If part of you is still caught in a diet mentality, and you are eating foods you think you "should" be eating, you may not be choosing satisfying foods. Discovering what you love and what truly pleases you is a powerful metaphor for the opportunity of midlife, right? Find what satisfies you and enjoy yourself. Trust your body to let you know when you've had enough. Remember to take small steps, as this takes time.

- *Cravings are information*: Don't be afraid of cravings. Diet culture makes you think in a binary of good and bad foods, but they are not good or bad; try to see them as neutral data. Cravings are your guide toward what will satisfy you. It takes courage to say "yes" to your cravings. Take your time and add a few new foods each week. Trust yourself here and do what works best for you.

- *Don't save the best until the end*: Saving your favorites until the end of the meal means you eat everything else to get to them, and you may push past the point of fullness. For example, if you have a yummy grilled sandwich before you and the gooey, melted middle is your favorite part, have that yummy part first. Then, you can be more discerning about how much of the rest of the sandwich you are interested in.
- *It's okay to be snobby*: You may notice that when you permit yourself to eat what satisfies you, you become more curious about what you genuinely enjoy and want to eat. This process may surprise you. Previously forbidden foods may not taste as good as you thought they would. You may feel overwhelmed when you give yourself more permission to eat the foods you love. Many clients go through an "I don't know what I want to eat!" phase. It is okay to eat "fancy" food if it is accessible. This is your chance to explore and discover what you love—another midlife metaphor. This is the perfect time to stop wasting yourself on anything that does not bring you satisfaction and support you in feeling well.

Habituation is real

What does "habituation" mean? Habituation refers to the process of allowing yourself a previously forbidden food and becoming used to it, so that you no longer find the food so enticing. It may feel like the food has power over you; this is the process of taking the power out of the food and giving it to yourself.

For example, if you do not allow yourself to eat chocolate chip cookies but then permit them as part of your disentangling from diet culture, you may fear that you will only eat chocolate chip cookies until you feel sick. And you might do that at first! Over time, the cookies become no big deal; you will only want them occasionally or lose interest in them for a while.

The same goes for any other previously forbidden foods. What if you are afraid to open a bag of your favorite chips because you believe you will eat them all? Now imagine if you decide to have a handful of chips with your lunch every single day. At some point, do you think you will start to want something other than chips until you realize chips are "no biggie!"? Many of my clients report feeling deeply empowered when throwing out the ice cream out because it has been in the freezer for so long that it has crystals!

Fullness and body respect

When you start to nourish yourself based on your internal wisdom rather than external rules, you will become increasingly aware of your hunger with time, practice, and effort. In my experience, fullness is more subtle and challenging to notice. *Noticing your fullness requires you to listen more intently, as if hearing a whisper from your body.*

Listening to your body's hunger sensations requires you to slow down and savor your food with fewer distractions. I recommend choosing a meal or snack most days to use as a chance to practice noticing your hunger and fullness. You may want to create stopping points during your eating to take a break, check in, and assess your level of fullness using the Hunger–Fullness Scale. (At some point, the Hunger–Fullness Scale will live in your head!) Check in at the halfway point, and if you are still hungry, eat a little more, then check again with another quarter of the food remaining. Practice, practice, practice!

This practice is more accessible if you can create quiet around you with few distractions and, hopefully, plenty of time. It is almost impossible if you feel rushed or distracted by a screen. Please be patient; noticing your fullness sensations may take time. I have a story illustrating how practicing a new skill like this works.

First practice in a more controlled environment to develop the skill of connecting with your body so that you receive your body's fullness signals. You can then try to sense your fullness with more noise around you, like eating with others. Please be patient; noticing your fullness sensations may take time and practice. There is no need for perfection or going fast here. Shooting for sometimes is good enough!

Of course, this is not a linear process. You will have days when you feel comfortable and confident with your ability to nourish yourself based on your body's wisdom. Then, you may have a more stressful or challenging period where you feel you've lost touch with your body and process. Healing and recovery do not happen in a straight line. *Give yourself some grace when you've dropped the thread.* You can begin again and find yourself right where you left off.

Curiosity as your antidote to judgment

Judgment is one of the most unhealthy qualities in a relationship. When you are judgmental in your relationship with your body, you ultimately reduce your self-worth. Please remember that you learned to do this, which was protective initially. Let's return to Robin's story.

Robin learned that a thinner body translated to approval and admiration based on her father's comments, her stepmother's comments and actions, and her pediatrician's comments. She learned that she would be safe from the harsh judgment of others if she made her body thinner. So, a part of her still tries to protect her even now. While she was learning the harms of manipulating her eating and activity in an effort to shrink her body, a part of her still judged her body as not thin enough, not good enough, not enough. This judgmental part was rooted in her early experiences, and that part still showed up to protect her from the judgment of others.

If you slow down and become curious about the source of your judgmental thoughts, you will likely notice their protective roots.

Harsh body judgment, which involves negative, critical, or dismissive attitudes, erodes a healthy relationship with your body. So, by putting effort into being curious when you notice your body-shaming thoughts, you have an opportunity to see where these thoughts are coming from and how they may have served you at once but no longer do. Curiosity supports mending your relationship with your body. A healthy relationship with your body thrives on body respect, compassion, and curiosity that is working toward more understanding.

When we're curious, we're more open to exploring and understanding different perspectives, which helps us move away from snap judgments, preconceived notions, and old, well-worn patterns. Instead of immediately categorizing something as right or wrong, good or bad, curiosity encourages you to ask questions, seek more profound understanding, and appreciate your self-talk's complexities, patterns, and resulting feelings.

The openness resulting from curiosity fosters empathy, reduces biases against food, eating, movement, and your body, and cultivates a more nuanced view of your experience. In many ways, curiosity can counteract the adverse effects of judgment by promoting a mindset of exploration, learning more about yourself, and opening the door to healing self-compassion.

Becoming curious opens up a connection with your body that supports body respect.

Body connection and consent asking

Another aspect of this mending process is asking for consent in your body relationship. I know that sounds weird, but let's break it down. I am not just referring to asking for permission when I say consent.

"Consent" derives from the Latin verb *consentīre*, which means "to share or join in a sensation or feeling, be in agreement or harmony." In this way, while checking with your body, you must be attuned to how your body is feeling with a little more curiosity. Consent asking can be a subtle process that moves toward you being more in sync with your body's need for fuel, movement, rest, pleasure, and satisfaction.

Consider Betty Martin, author of *The Art of Receiving and Giving: The Wheel of Consent*, who describes consent as having four quadrants; Taking, Allowing, Giving, and Receiving. I am going to translate her quadrants into how you are relating with your body.

Taking

Taking what your body needs in the form of rest, play, pleasure, or nourishment may be an act that is incredibly uncomfortable for you. Acknowledging your needs is a vulnerable process. This may be especially hard for you if, as a child, you felt you needed to care for others to feel safe and valued. It may also feel emotionally risky to let others see your needs. It may be hard for you to enjoy yummy foods, rest, or play in front of others.

Allowing

This requires being aware of and discerning your body's wants and needs along with your body's limits. What do you want to eat? Sometimes this question is a surprisingly challenging one if you've been caught up in food rules for years. What do you need to eat to feel the way you want? For example, if you want to feel energized, what food appeals to you? Or, if you want to feel comforted, what appeals? How much is enough? How much is too much? You get to explore and discover your body's preferences and limits. This requires mindfulness and curiosity and can be playful. This may create more generosity in how you relate to your body and even your ability to relax and begin to trust yourself.

Giving (serving)

This is usually where we are most comfortable and familiar. We are accustomed to providing the nourishment or movement we think we "should" give our bodies. Usually, we are more confident in relating to our bodies as our responsibility. We are more accustomed to serving our bodies and expecting that our bodies will serve us in return.

Receiving (accepting)

This may be a little uncomfortable or scary. Receiving your attention is required, which can be a new and unfamiliar experience. Some feel they just don't know how to receive their own care and attention. With time and practice, this supports a healthy relationship with your body.

What does this look like in an experience?

Lillian's story

One of my clients, Lillian, was in a rush one morning and grabbed a bar on her way out the door with the intention of eating it on her way to work. She thought she was doing the right thing for her body because at least she wasn't skipping breakfast.

She reached for the breakfast bar as she drove down the road, feeling like she was on "automatic pilot." But as she was opening the bar, she started a conversation with her body. She asked herself, "Is this what I really want this morning? Will this satisfy me? Will this support and sustain me this morning?" The answer to each inquiry was a resounding "No!" so she put the bar back in its wrapper, saving it for another time, and stopped to grab a more sustaining and yummy breakfast sandwich.

As she told this story, she was excited to report that she 1) was shocked that she had a conversation with her body, 2) felt much more respectful of her body, almost like she had a "new friend," and 3) actually felt more comfortable and confident in her body. She was astounded at all this and felt like she had made a huge step, although she felt it was "a silly thing to do."

I affirmed that this was indeed a big deal in that she:

1 Felt connected with her body
2 Was listening to her body's disinterest in the bar
3 Checked in (Consent) with her body and discovered that this bar would not support her
4 Took action to meet her body's needs.

The result was feeling a closer relationship with her body, which was a pleasant surprise and a "win" to be celebrated!

Diet and fitness culture taught you to ride roughshod over your body, ignoring signals that let you know that you are tired and need a break, that you are craving food with a more preferred taste, something other than what you "should" eat, something more sustaining. Having a connection with your body that allows you to notice when your body is making a request is in and of itself a big step and a major win!

Whenever you check in with your body and ask for consent as you make choices about nourishment, movement, rest, or taking a break, you honor and respect your body as a valid partner. This is precisely how you rebuild and mend your relationship with your body. You'll find more about consent in the Resources section.

Rebuilding trust in your body sounds challenging. It is. You will make mistakes and mess up. So, the most essential ingredient is Self-Compassion.

Self-compassion is essential

Learning to give yourself plenty of compassion is essential when challenging limiting beliefs and old patterns that no longer serve you, healing body relationship wounds, and changing your mindset and behaviors. How you handle messing up can make all the difference in your ability to keep going. With a kinder and more accepting attitude, you are more likely to learn from your mistakes and have the stamina to keep going rather than give up.

So what is self-compassion exactly?

Self-compassion is being kind, understanding, and supportive toward yourself, especially when you make mistakes. You are not alone if this feels false, cheesy, or uncomfortable. Most of my clients say that practicing self-compassion is one of the hardest aspects of their healing process. My theory is that we feel vulnerable when we are kind to ourselves because it feels like we are "letting our guard down," so to speak.

Sadly, we've learned to be hard on ourselves and push harder, believing that we will be more "successful" by being harsher in the tone we take with ourselves. But in fact, the opposite is true. Being more self-critical when you make a mistake actually makes you feel more shame, which in turn makes you feel more uncomfortable, which does not encourage you to keep going.

I know clients are progressing well when they tell me they are not beating themselves up as much as they once did. Progress!

So, where to begin? Kristen Neff (2003) has extensively researched self-compassion and describes the three main ingredients of a self-compassion practice.

1 *Mindfulness*: Being aware of your thoughts and feelings in the present moment without judgment. Acknowledge your thoughts and feelings, such as this is hard, or this sucks, and name what you are experiencing without identifying with your emotions. So acknowledging that you messed up does not mean you ARE a mess.
2 *Shared humanity*: Recognizing that we all make mistakes, struggle, face challenges, and feel pain. It is part of being human. You are not broken or a mess when you mess up.
3 *Self-kindness*: Instead of being overly critical or harsh when you make mistakes, offer yourself kindness, understanding, and encouragement.

If this feels overwhelming and you think, "I don't know how to do this," embarking on a self-compassion practice can feel like learning a new language. It often helps to think of how you would treat a friend or your younger self if they messed up. Then, apply the same sentiments and words to yourself. Perhaps keep a photograph of yourself as a child where you will see it often, such as on your phone or laptop, as a screensaver. This reminder of yourself as a child usually helps you soften how you speak to yourself when working on self-compassion practices. Let's give it a try.

Self-compassion practice

My favorite self-compassion practices are adapted from those I learned from Jack Kornfield and Sharon Salzberg over many years of study and practice, both for personal and professional reasons. I would call myself a "recovering perfectionist," a trait I share with the majority of my clients.

Begin by making yourself as comfortable as possible. You can do this practice in any position you find yourself in—lying down, seated, or standing. Please be generous and support yourself with blankets or pillows that help you feel as comfortable as possible.

You can close your eyes or leave them open, your gaze soft and resting in front of you. Scan your body for any places where you are holding tension or bracing and see if you can soften and let go any amount. If you are comfortable connecting with your breath, you can also check in and notice the nature of your breath, reminding yourself that you can trust your body to breathe.

Bring into your mind's eye the image of a being in your life whose love is uncomplicated. Notice how your care for them bubbles up easily, without effort, when you picture them there. Notice any changes in bodily sensations you may experience as you think of them. Is there warmth around your heart, an easy, soft smile on your face, or a crinkling around your eyes? Take a few moments to notice and allow yourself to feel these sensations.

You may also hold yourself as a child in your mind's eye.

As you look into your beloved's eyes, remember the burdens they carry. Take note of the struggles, the confusion, the pain, the grief, and the frustrations they've experienced. Notice what happens within you as you consider their pain and suffering. Notice how easily tenderness and care bubble up for you as you consider their hardships. Allow yourself to feel the bodily sensations that accompany your love and care. Then say to your beloved:

> May you be held in compassion.
> May your pain and suffering be eased.
> May you live with a peaceful heart.

Then, notice them looking back at you as they consider your pain, suffering, frustrations, confusion, and struggles. Allow yourself to receive the love and tenderness they feel for you as they consider your hardships. It can be hard to receive love and kindness from others, so if you are experiencing resistance here, **hold your resistance with care and compassion**. Remind yourself that resistance is usually rooted in part of you feeling vulnerable and needing to protect yourself. Do you notice bodily sensations as you receive kindness and compassion from a beloved or your younger self? If so, allow yourself to feel these sensations. Hear your beloved say to you:

> May you be held in compassion.
> May your pain and suffering be eased.
> May you live with a peaceful heart.

Now, for the final step in this process, take this care, compassion, and kindness and offer it to yourself. Consider your struggles, frustrations, pain, grief, confusion, and suffering. Can you find the same care and tenderness and offer it to yourself? Say to yourself:

> May I be held in compassion.
> May my pain and suffering be eased.
> May I live with a peaceful heart.

Please repeat this as many times as you need to. Notice any shifting and changing in your body and around your heart. Is there a softening or a bracing at any particular place? Allow yourself to notice without judgment, and with compassionate curiosity.

Take your time and slowly let this go as you return to your day.

It may be helpful to journal about what you notice with this practice.

I highly recommend that you commit to self-compassion practices in your life. A frequent, if not daily, self-compassion practice will help you more successfully mend your relationship with food, eating, and your body. Self-compassion practices are well-researched and documented to benefit your well-being.

Now that you are in the process of dismantling and ditching the rigid rules and deprivation of anti-diet/wellness and anti-aging/longevity culture, and your relationship with your body is on the mend (and you're more interested in caring for your body!), let's discuss the choices that support nourishing your vitality and well-being. If the idea of discussing foods that support your well-being midlife and beyond trigger your old patterns of judgment and rigidity, please skip the next chapter. Remember that you are the expert of you. Take what is helpful and leave the rest.

6

Nourishing your body for vitality and well-being

This chapter includes specific recommendations for meeting your body's needs in midlife, free of diet culture and restrictions, by adopting an *additive* attitude. We'll discuss adding particular aspects of nourishment, such as hydration, fiber, specific nutrients like calcium, and the importance of enough protein balanced with carbohydrates and fats. This chapter promotes *adding* foods to your diet and the concept that satisfaction is essential to being well-nourished.

Before we get into more of the nuts and bolts of wise nutrition in midlife and beyond, please remember:

- You are the expert of you. I know nutrition, but I don't know you!
- You are unique, and so are your needs.
- Our culture's over-focus and reductive approach to food and eating makes nutrition seem much more complicated than it needs to be.
- General recommendations will meet your needs and protect you from overthinking and feeling anxious about what you eat.
- Your body is for you to enjoy, and eating food can also be for your pleasure!
- What is the most common mistake women in midlife and beyond make with their diets? Not eating enough and being undernourished!

Normal eating

Did you ever feel "normal" about your eating?

The older I get, the more I believe there is no such thing as normal. Normal is a setting on the washing machine, as they say. However, when I was in grad school in the 80s, I read studies about the effect of chronic restriction using control groups of subjects who were "normal eaters" or those not exposed to diet culture. *That type of research is no longer possible because of the ubiquitous nature of diet culture.* Let that sink in.

I miss sitting down to share a meal and never hearing a comment about food, body worries, rules, or guilt. When we discuss our food rules or worries over a meal, we may be bonding over our common source of pain and struggle. If you grew up hearing judgment about food, eating, and bodies, this may feel "automatic" for you. It's complicated and challenging to create a flexible and relaxed approach to eating. Sometimes, I think we've all been brainwashed by diet/wellness culture, and anti-aging messages aren't helping either!

If you feel like you don't even know what "normal eating" looks like anymore, I offer you a reference point that many of my clients find helpful. Try the following for a definition of *normal eating:*

- Normal eating ... is going to the table hungry, and eating until you are satisfied.
- Normal eating ... is being able to choose food you enjoy and to eat it and truly get enough of it—not just stop eating because you think you should.
- Normal eating ... is being able to give some thought to your food selection so you get nutritious food, but not being so wary and restrictive that you miss out on enjoyable food.
- Normal eating ... is giving yourself permission to eat because you are happy, sad, or bored, or just because it feels good.

- Normal eating ... is mostly three meals a day—or four or five—or it can be choosing to munch along the way.
- Normal eating ... is leaving cookies on the plate because you will let yourself have cookies again tomorrow, or eating more now because they taste so great!
- Normal eating ... is overeating at times, and feeling stuffed and uncomfortable ... and undereating at times, and wishing you had more.
- Normal eating ... is trusting your body to make up for your mistakes in eating.
- Normal eating ... takes up some of your time and attention, but keeps its place as only one important area of your life.

In short, normal eating is flexible. It varies in response to hunger, schedule, food, access, and feelings.

-Ellyn Satter of the Ellyn Satter Institute

The hallmarks of "normal" eating are:

- Flexibility
- Little to no guilt or anxiety related to food and eating
- No calculations or counting
- No need to compensate for what you ate
- Led mainly by data from the body, such as feeling satisfied
- Permission for pleasure
- Able to engage with valued aspects of living your life free of intrusive thoughts about food and eating
- Being present with your experience and to others when you are eating.

Anti-aging and diet/wellness cultures have normalized disordered eating and tell you that your midlife+ body is broken and needs to be fixed. This undermines your relationship with your body, and makes it confusing and challenging to nourish yourself with a relaxed, flexible, and "normal-eating" mindset.

You are simply trying to do the right thing based on the dominant messages you are receiving from anti-aging and diet/wellness culture. It is easy to find yourself stuck in these patterns without realizing what is happening because this is so normalized! Please be gentle with yourself and give yourself some grace.

Within these pages, I'm committed to helping you find your sweet spot and eat to feel vital and sustained while making choices that give you pleasure and satisfy you!

An additive attitude

I've been researching evidence-based recommendations about nourishing your body to support your well-being in midlife and beyond since I pivoted to this specialty in 2019 when I turned 60. The nutrition recommendations I'm giving you is vetted to be *free of diet/wellness culture mess*. That means it's focused on choices you can *add* to your diet to support your well-being rather than food rules that contribute to you feeling deprived or concerned about your weight.

Overall, it is true that *regardless of your efforts*, aging and the body changes that come with it happen! Changes in your lifecycle and stressors, diseases, medications, sleep, and hormones all impact your body. Aging changes your nutritional needs because your body's metabolism, composition, and cellular function shift as you get older. Accepting this and working with these changes rather than denying, avoiding, or fighting these truths is essential.

Before we get into it, I want to emphasize that my priority is helping you feel joyful and more relaxed about food again! Our culture has reduced the bounty of the food on our planet to nutrition facts. We are overwhelmingly out of balance when it comes to food and nutrition, fueled by anti-fat bias, classism, and a moral panic about body weight. Yes, I am a Registered Dietitian/Nutritionist and want to support your well-being. But I've been sitting across from the pain and struggle that develop when we lose our balance for decades! What I offer here is an attempt to right the ship. You *can* savor and find pleasure in the foods you love without the fallout of guilt and thoughts of compensation.

Don't forget to hydrate

Considering the long list of reasons to stay hydrated, keep your water bottle filled and within reach. According to Harvard's School of Public Health, water:

- Maintains body temperature
- Lubricates your joints
- Prevents infections
- Delivers nutrients to your cells
- Keeps your organs functioning properly
- Improves sleep quality
- Elevates your mood
- Boosts cognition.

The consequences of inadequate hydration are also related to the function of your brain. Our brains are highly vascular, meaning there is a great deal of blood flow, so the integrity of our blood affects our brains first and foremost. Being less hydrated means you are more likely to experience fatigue, irritability, reduced cognitive functioning, and headaches. You've probably heard that before, so why aren't we motivated to drink more water? This might be a good time to take a sip of water 😊

According to recent research, as we age, we become less sensitive to changes in our blood, signifying that we are becoming dehydrated. We simply do not become thirsty when we could use a glass of water to keep our blood in tip-top shape. So, we need to get in the habit of drinking water throughout the day regardless of thirst. The amount of water recommended each day is still around 8 glasses (8 oz) of water.

To stay hydrated, you can also drink tea or other water-containing beverages and eat foods high in water, such as soup, cucumbers, and watermelon. All of these count toward meeting your daily needs.

The role of carbohydrates: or how not to be a b*tch

When I think about carbohydrates, I think about a science lesson from elementary school.

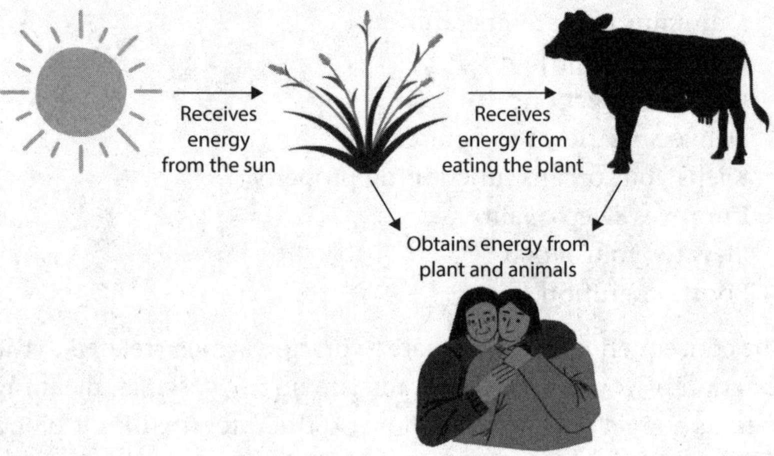

I interpret this and translate it to my clients because we consume power from the sun when we eat plants. The primary source of carbohydrates in our diet is plants. So my question is, how can you possibly worry about eating sunshine?

One of the dominant themes in diet/wellness culture is limiting, managing, controlling, and avoiding carbohydrates. This theme is even more pronounced in the Meno-sphere, a term I use to describe wellness influencers focused on (or preying on) women in midlife. The echo chamber of the meno-sphere constantly says eating carbs will mean more belly fat. The fear-mongering continues from there with the story that belly fat will cause insulin resistance and chronic diseases.

In fact, your blood sugar is managed by complicated feedback and counter-feedback loops because your body's design is amazing! Your body's capacity to manage your blood sugar and remain disease-free depends on many complex factors:

- Genetic predisposition
- Stress
- Sleep quality
- Environmental stressors
- Medication (some medications impair glucose metabolism, such as steroids)
- Movement
- Hormonal imbalances, such as PCOS
- Aging (your pancreas understandably changes with use and over time)
- Gestational diabetes
- Smoking
- Alcohol use
- Low fiber diet
- There is some speculation that viruses, such as Covid-19, can tip the scales toward developing diabetes.

Reread the above and notice:

- Eating sugar or carbohydrates is NOT ON THIS LIST!

I hope you notice that *adding* more fiber (we'll get into this more later), movement, high-quality sleep, stress management, smoking cessation, and avoiding alcohol have a far more significant influence on your health than belly fat. Perhaps the focus on belly fat, which is a very normal and ever-changing part of a woman's body, is actually due to patriarchy, unrealistic beauty ideals, and weight stigma. Just saying.

I have a t-shirt from the outstanding dietitian Anna Sweeney that says, "You're Nicer With Carbs." So true! Your brain's preferred fuel is carbohydrates, specifically glucose, AKA sugar.

You know what it feels like when your blood sugar starts to drop, right? The word "hangry" was created for a reason!

Your brain depends on the delivery of glucose from your diet. Carbohydrates are the most abundant nutrient on the planet, but your body stores very little glycogen, which is how your body stores glucose for easy access. Remember our discussion of the Minnesota Starvation Experiment earlier and the symptoms noted in the subjects when they were undernourished.

There are significant consequences to your brain's preferred fuel supply dropping. Common symptoms are:

- Feeling shaky or jittery
- Cold, clammy sweat that may come on suddenly
- Feeling dizzy, light-headed, faint, or like you might pass out
- Intense hunger or a sudden, urgent need to eat
- Dull or throbbing headache that can come on quickly
- Brain fog or confusion
- Suddenly feeling anxious, nervous, irritable, or angry
- Heart palpitations
- Sudden and unexplained fatigue or weakness
- Blurry or double-vision
- Numbness or tingling, especially in your extremities.

Does this list remind you of anything? It is eerily similar to the list of symptoms often attributed to perimenopause or menopause. Maybe our carb restrictions, a common recommendation in reaction to the changes in our bodies during perimenopause, are making our perimenopause/menopause symptoms even worse.

Some people receive early warning signs and notice more subtle sensations, such as irritability and fatigue. Some experience more extreme symptoms if they missed the more subtle signals early on. In my experience, those who've lived through deprivation and restriction due to food insecurity, an eating disorder, or chronic dieting are more likely to experience these symptoms of low blood sugar. It seems the body is working to protect you from experiencing the threat of being undernourished again and does not tolerate getting too hungry by sending these urgent messages, translated to "Please nourish me, NOW!"

Carbohydrates are also a source of great pleasure. They are associated with social gatherings and celebrations and are often a token of love and affection. Consider the significance of the phrase "breaking bread together." The times we connect with our beloveds and ourselves usually include food, specifically carbohydrates. Over the years, countless clients have told me that eating foods high in carbohydrates makes them feel better in so many ways:

- Grounded
- Calmer
- Soothed
- Contented.

At the same time, the loud message from both anti-aging/longevity and diet/wellness cultures is that eating carbohydrates is "bad" for you, in a word. This long-standing message has seeped into our cultural lexicon. Think of the language we use when describing foods high in carbohydrates: "sinful," "a cheat treat," "tempting," "naughty," "worth it," "a splurge," and "decadent." If you didn't know we were talking about food, you might think we were describing a moral transgression because that is how diet culture leaves you relating to foods that create pleasure with guilt and shame.

I am not saying, "Just eat everything you want." Instead, I am saying that you should allow yourself to eat a variety of foods, including those that bring you pleasure and satisfaction and the foods you love, enjoy, and support a greater sense of well-being in your life. With those foods, you are more likely to stop eating when you are satisfied. If you are *not* satisfied, you are much more likely to experience a reactive binge-eating episode or continue to eat until you are overfull.

I know this is difficult if you've been dieting and believe you cannot be trusted around the foods you love. You may go through an initial phase of eating only the foods you've been deprived of.

Your body will eventually habituate and stabilize with your discernment on board. Remember what you learned earlier about mending your relationship with your body. Eating a variety of foods, including those you love, is the culmination of this process, which is to be celebrated!

A meal including a combination of carbohydrates, protein, and fat supports you in reaching satiety. Experiencing satisfaction and slowing down enough to notice your satiety encourages you to stop when you've had enough. No more calculating, counting, and tracking is needed! Trusting your body invites true liberation from diet culture.

Protein and proteinmania

Our obsession with the protein in our diets is at an all-time high. And this is especially true for those in midlife and beyond. Any product with the phrase "high-protein" is automatically anointed with a wellness halo. According to Forbes Health (Davis, 2024), "TikTok data shows #highprotein scored a whopping 2 billion U.S. views over the last 12 months" as of February 2024.

There is no question that the macronutrient protein is essential. I'm sure you've heard that protein is crucial in your body as the primary "building block" for all your cells and tissues. More specifically, protein plays a role in:

- Repair following injury and illness
- Formation of hormones (your body's messengers)
- Formation of enzymes (your body's catalysts for digestion, muscle contraction, blood clotting, metabolism of energy)
- The balance of pH and fluid
- The structural component of your muscle mass and other structures, such as collagen

- Being a potential energy source
- Transporting nutrients such as oxygen to every cell of your body via your blood
- Immune system function.

Considering protein's crucial role in your well-being, remember that your body cannot manufacture protein; therefore, you must include it in your diet.

The role of protein in our diets in midlife and beyond is even more vital. A growing body of evidence supports the benefits of including more protein in our diets for those 50 and older. We lose muscle mass as we get older no matter what, but including more protein in our diets and strength training will slow this loss.

Another significant benefit of including protein in meals and snacks is improved blood sugar management. Combined with fiber, this slows your body's digestion, absorption, and metabolism of the foods you eat, delaying the rise in your blood sugar.

Yet, with all of this legitimate interest in including protein in your diet, I will boldly not recommend how many grams of protein you should eat! Gasp! I am confident you have calculated this number based on multiple recommendations, which range widely, most of them excessively high. The conversation about how much protein we need has taken on an intensity that parallels religion and politics. My stance is that nutrition is based on science, not opinions. Therefore, I do not recommend that you follow the recommendations of wellness influencers on social media.

You can do a beautiful job of meeting your body's needs without counting, calculating, and tracking grams of protein. As I explained in Chapter 2, tracking and counting anything about your food removes you from your experience and contributes to potential worry and obsession. Including foods that contain significant amounts of protein in the majority of your meals and snacks will meet your needs. I experimented with this notion with my diet and those clients who wished to share their eating journals with me and found this to be the case most of the time.

With just a bit of intention to include protein in your meals and snacks, you will successfully meet your needs—and avoid getting caught up in the high-protein frenzy. To do this, you must understand where protein can be found in your food supply. So, let's take a look at protein sources.

Plant proteins were once considered lesser quality than animal proteins based on incomplete amino acids, but that has been refuted in recent years. Christopher Gardner, a professor of medicine at Stanford University, discovered that all plant protein sources—from peanuts to edamame beans—contain all essential amino acids. Admittedly, they contain smaller concentrations of amino acids than protein from animal sources, but if you eat a variety of foods, this is not something to worry about.

Plant proteins offer additional nutrients, such as fiber, which supports your gut health. Case in point: eating foods provides greater benefits than supplements, and many foods include some protein, which adds up throughout the day. For example, you may not think of oatmeal or whole-grain bread when considering protein, but a serving may contain 4–5 grams.

A plant protein is protein that comes from plant-based sources rather than animal products. These proteins are found in foods like beans, nuts, seeds, and wholegrains.

Plant Protein

• 4 oz. firm tofu	18 g
• 2/3 C shelled edamame	11 g
• 3 oz. tempeh	17 g
• 1/2 C lentils, cooked	12 g
• 1/2 C chickpeas, cooked	8 g
• 1/2 C black beans, cooked	8 g

- 1 C quinoa, cooked   8 g
- 2 T peanut butter   7 g
- 1 oz. peanuts   7g
- 1 oz. almonds   7 g
- ¼ C pumpkin seeds   9 g
- ⅓ C hummus   5 g
- 3 T hemp hearts   10 g
- 2 T chia seeds   5 g
- ¾ C bean flour pasta   14 g
- 1 large oyster mushroom   5 g
- Serving soy/pea protein powder   24 g

Animal Protein

- 1 oz. beef, poultry, pork   7 g
- 1 oz. seafood   7 g
- I egg   7 g
- 1 C 2% milk   8 g
- 1 C lowfat greek yogurt   20 g
- ½ C cottage cheese   12 g
- 1 oz. most cheeses   7 g

So a day of you meeting your protein needs might look like this:

First meal

1 C Greek yogurt (or plant-based yogurt)
3 T hemp hearts
2 T chia seeds
Fruit
Latte made with 1 C cow's milk (or soy milk)

Second meal

Sandwich: 2 oz. turkey/1 oz. cheese on whole grain bread
At least ⅓ C hummus plus veggies

Vegetarian alternative: 1 C lentils, edamame or tofu added to salad with pumpkin seeds
Whole grain crackers

Afternoon snack

At least 2 oz. dark chocolate dusted almonds

Third meal

4 oz. poultry, meat, seafood, or tofu
Starch
Veggie

Evening snack

Your choice

The above shoots for the high side, well exceeding 100 grams, just for the sake of this experiment. I have only included portions for the protein sources here for the purpose of illustration. I hope this is reassuring that you:

- Don't need to purchase special powders and bars. You certainly can if you wish! The emphasis here is that you have choices
- Can find these meals/snacks to be satisfying and sustainable
- Don't need to stress about the protein grams you eat.

If these protein servings are too large for you, consider a smoothie made with a protein powder or a high-protein bar as your afternoon snack.

Remember, skipping meals makes it unlikely that you will meet your protein needs.

Befriending fat in your food

How you think about fat in your diet may be traced back to the fat-free food craze of the 1980s. It all started with research published in the 50s, which was then adopted by the American Heart Association (AHA) in the 60s and further defined by the AHA in the 70s. In the 80s, the US government made similar recommendations more broadly, followed by the food industry's spread of low-fat and fat-free diet products and recommendations from popular media. The recommendations to restrict dietary fat were based on concerns about the prevalence of cardiovascular disease and the diet–heart hypothesis. This hypothesis posed that diets high in saturated fats and cholesterol significantly cause cardiovascular disease.

I was in graduate school studying nutritional science in the mid-80s and was on the receiving end of this ideology. The benefits of a low-fat diet had a significant hold on the mindset of Western culture with four cultural nutrition myths (La Berge, 2008):

- The American tradition of low-calorie, low-fat diets for weight reduction
- The diet–heart hypothesis dating from the post-World War II era
- The politics of food and low fat
- The promotion of low fat by the popular health media.

By the late 1990s and early 2000s, research indicated some fats, including avocados, olive oil, nuts, seeds, nut butters, and fatty fish, showed health benefits. Even eggs found redemption! As a consumer of nutritional guidance, you may have experienced whiplash as the "recommendations" began to shift and change.

Another not-so-small factor to consider is that some vitamins, vitamins A, D, and E, are fat-soluble. Fat in your diet helps the body absorb these vitamins.

Replacing saturated fats with polyunsaturated fats is well-documented to lower the risk of developing cardiovascular disease. Monounsaturated fats are also a good choice and can be found primarily in olive and avocado oils. The only fats the human body requires are omega-3 fatty acids (EPA & DHA) from fatty fish or fish/algae supplements and omega-6 fatty acids from nuts, seeds, avocadoes, canola, rapeseed, soybean, sunflower, and safflower oils. In a typical diet, it's far easier to get enough omega-6 than omega-3; supplementation may be beneficial. Please check with your healthcare provider to discuss this decision.

Quick reminder:

- Saturated fats have a particular chemical composition that makes them solid at room temperature. Most saturated fats come from animal food sources, but some plant oils, such as palm and coconut oil, also contain high levels.
- Polyunsaturated fats are typically liquid at room temperature but start to turn solid when chilled. Examples include canola, corn, soybean and sunflower oils.
- Monounsaturated fats are similar to polyunsaturated fats with a little different chemical make-up and are also typically liquid at room temperature but start to turn solid when chilled. Olive oil is probably the most well-known example. Avocados and peanuts are also high in monounsaturated fats.

An often-forgotten fact is that your body has the ability to regulate its cholesterol status. When your dietary cholesterol intake is very low, your body increases gut absorption and cholesterol synthesis. When your dietary cholesterol intake is high, your body suppresses synthesis and increases excretion. However, genetic inheritance may alter your body's ability to regulate blood cholesterol levels. Lifestyle changes may not be sufficient to control your cholesterol, specifically LDL cholesterol if you have a genetic predisposition for high LDL cholesterol. LDL cholesterol is a type of cholesterol that transports cholesterol from your liver out into your bloodstream and potentially accumulates in arteries as plaque which contributes to cardiovascular and other diseases. I recommend speaking with your healthcare provider to discuss management through your lifestyle and possible medication needs.

The rise of the Mediterranean diet provided most healthcare providers with a common-sense place to land. The Mediterranean diet is known for its abundance of fruits, vegetables and legumes, whole grains, along with fat from extra virgin olive oil, nuts, seeds, and avocado. It recommends protein sources like lean protein from fish, poultry, and eggs with moderate amounts of red meat, along with moderate amounts of dairy products. Spices and seasonings from garlic, onion, oregano, cumin, and other flavorful ingredients are encouraged. The Mediterranean Diet shifted the focus from low total fat to low saturated fat intake, encouraging monounsaturated fats in the diet. A diet high in red meat, cheese, and butter (saturated fat) such as the carnivore diet is not recommended for heart and brain health.

The concern about our blood cholesterol levels is not limited to preventing cardiovascular disease. A growing body of research, including the 2024 update of Lancet's Commission on Dementia (Livingston et al., 2024), associates our brain health with our blood cholesterol levels. Higher blood levels of LDL-cholesterol, ApoB and lower levels of HDL-cholesterol increase our risk for a decline in brain function as we age.

Therefore, I want to highlight this topic. ApoB is a protein that binds to LDL-cholesterol and plays a role in the transport of cholesterol in the bloodstream. HDL-cholesterol is considered the good guy of cholesterols because it plays a crucial role in removing excess cholesterol from the bloodstream and preventing its accumulation in the arteries. A complex interplay of factors beyond diet, including genetics, movement, stress, hormones, smoking, medications, and disease processes, influences cholesterol levels. If you are concerned about your lab values, I recommend speaking with your healthcare provider about your specific lab results and your overall health and lifestyle.

Including monounsaturated and polyunsaturated fats in your meals and snacks has benefits. Fat slows the digestion and absorption of the nutrients in your food, helping to manage your blood sugar and offering more satiety for a longer time. Fat in your food also dramatically increases flavor, pleasure, and satisfaction.

For example, if you are eating a very low or non-fat snack, such as pretzels or dry popcorn, you will likely only be able to stop eating once you feel overly full due to the low potential for satiety. Suppose you have a snack that is very satisfying and contains fat and protein, such as nuts or nut butter with fruit. In that case, you will likely feel satisfied and be able to stop eating when you notice you are satisfied, which is far more empowering and comfortable.

When you start to make choices about your eating with the intention to feel satisfied, experiencing pleasure, and feeling energized, vital, and sustained, you will likely make choices that mix carbohydrates, fat, and protein *without* spending much time in your head making calculations. You can trust yourself, your instincts, and your body to handle this decision-making process. What a freeing experience!

Friendly reminder and body break

This is another friendly reminder that we are walking a fine line here! We are trying to balance making choices that support you in being free of diet culture and supporting feeling well in midlife and beyond. This has the potential to feel overwhelming.

This book is dedicated to helping you care for your body without compromising your emotional health and spirit. It is a fine art, but you can find your sweet spot. Remember your self-compassion practice, be flexible with this, and please let go of trying to be perfect! The goal of "good enough" works best!

It may be time to check in with yourself and take a break. Are you starting to experience more connection with your body and the echoes accompanying your body breaks?

Special note to those who are feeling resistant to the information in this chapter. I see you! Remember what I said earlier about resistance being a sign a part of you is feeling protective? If you've experienced chronic dieting, food trauma, or an eating disorder, hearing anything that comes close to a rule about your eating makes you want to run, push back, or shut down, I recommend that you acknowledge this wise protective part and decide if you want to skip this chapter or proceed with an abundance of self-compassion and caution.

The finer points—micronutrients and such

Let's look now at some other additions you can usefully bring into your diet.

Fiber

Remember when I talked about the introductory science lesson you probably learned in grade school about the sun being *the* energy source for your body? The other lesson you learned at school was that the big difference between animal and plant cells is that all plant cells have a cell wall. I know I'm very nerdy and love science, but I vividly remember these images of cells with and without cell walls on the chalkboard. It helps to remember that the cell wall of plants is not digestible by the human body and, therefore, is what we call fiber.

> Eating plants = Eating fiber

Dietary fiber serves several functions vital to your health and well-being. It plays a primary role in maintaining a healthy gut microbiome and digestion. Fiber-containing foods contain both soluble and insoluble fiber.

Soluble fibers bind to cholesterol in bile and prevent it from being reabsorbed into the bloodstream. Good soluble fiber sources include:

- Apples
- Bananas
- Berries
- Pears
- Avocados
- Potatoes
- Beans
- Lentils
- Tofu
- Edamame
- Oats
- Flax seeds.

Insoluble fiber promotes bowel regularity and prevents constipation, supports gut health, slows down digestion therefore increasing feelings of satiety, and helps to regulate your blood sugar. Good sources of insoluble fibers are similar to soluble as most plants contain both types of fiber. Excellent sources of insoluble fiber are:

- Fruits (e.g., apples, pears, berries)
- Vegetables (e.g., broccoli, cauliflower, peas)
- Whole grains (e.g., wheat bran, brown rice)
- Nuts and seeds (e.g., almonds, walnuts, flaxseed)
- Legumes (e.g., beans, lentils).

Including more plants for fiber carries the bonus of many other micronutrients! This is one of those old-school recommendations that stands the test of time. Eat more plants, especially the colorful ones that contain polyphenols. Polyphenols help fight oxidative stress, which results in illness. They are found in more colorful fruits and vegetables. The adage "eat the rainbow" stands as wise advice.

Choosing plants as a protein source several times a week has the added benefit of including sources of fiber and polyphenols, which may explain why more plant protein is associated with a reduced risk of cardiovascular disease. There is growing evidence that the same is valid for protecting cognitive function, dementia, and neurodegenerative diseases.

This time, I will give you a goal number to shoot for because fiber is rarely related to weight regulation, and meeting this goal requires your attention. It is also vital for your well-being to include adequate amounts of fiber in your diet.

Fiber intake

Aim for a minimum of 30 g of fiber daily. If you are not accustomed to this much fiber, start slowly to minimize gastrointestinal distress and build to your comfortable tolerance.

To meet this goal, here are some recommendations that may help you consider your daily/weekly choices. Remember, no need to be perfect! These are foods you can ADD to your diet.

• Leafy greens	3+ servings/day
• Colorful veggies	3+ servings/day
• Fruit	1–2+ servings/day
• Whole grains	3+ ½ C servings/day
• Beans	4+ ½ C servings/week
• Nuts/Seeds	~¼+ C serving/day
• Olive/Avocado oil	use as your preferred fats
• Omega-3 rich fish	1+ 3 oz. serving/week

If possible, include:

- Cruciferous veggies
- Alliums, such as onions and garlic
- Fermented foods
- Dark chocolate and cacao
- Avocados
- Tofu and edamame

B-vitamins

Around age 50, research shows that your gut does not absorb B vitamins as well, and this ability. It is also noteworthy that some medications interfere with the absorption of B-12, including common over-the-counter medications that lower stomach acids and Metformin, a medication often taken to manage blood glucose levels. Therefore, it is easy to find yourself with a deficiency in B-12 and B-6.

A deficiency in B-12 can cause anemia and neurological changes, such as tingling and numbness in your extremities and problems with balance. It can also cause confusion, brain fog, and can cause permanent damage to your nervous system (peripheral nerves, spinal cord, and brain) if left untreated. The tricky part is that these symptoms mimic many other symptoms of hormonal changes experienced in midlife+ so it is very important to be seen by a healthcare provider and have lab work done to check for deficiency.

Vitamin B-12 is found in animal products, so it can be challenging to meet your needs if you eat fewer animal products. Depending on what your lab work reveals, you may need to take a supplement or receive regular B-12 injections.

Deficiency in B-6 is also a concern as we age and can result in changes in cognitive function. B-6 is more readily available in our food supply and can also be found in supplement form. Again, discuss the need for supplementation with your healthcare provider.

Vitamin D

Vitamin D is crucial to your bone health, immune system function, and brain health. The best way to maintain a healthy vitamin D level is to be exposed to sunlight for short periods up to 15 minutes. Please consult with your dermatologist if you have concerns if this is best for your well-being.

However, your skin's ability to synthesize vitamin D decreases as you age, and vitamin D is fat soluble. Therefore, if you have digestive issues that create malabsorption of fat, such as celiac disease, Crohn's disease, or ulcerative colitis, you are likely unable to absorb vitamin D as well as you need to.

Vitamin D deficiency may play a role in:

- Poor immune function
- Cognitive decline
- Mood instability
- Decline in bone density
- Muscle health.

At the time of this writing, there is ongoing research and discussion of the role of Vitamin D in many other diseases, but they remain inconclusive. The most substantial evidence relates to bone health.

It is also challenging to meet our vitamin D needs from our food supply. Ask your healthcare provider to check your blood's vitamin D level. It is common to require dietary supplements to meet your body's needs for vitamin D. Please discuss this with your healthcare provider as your lab values will determine the best supplement dosage for you.

Vitamin K

Promising research suggests that vitamin K provides some defense against age-related conditions like osteoporosis, osteoarthritis, and cardiovascular disease. It is best known for its role in helping blood to clot, the essential process that helps the body reduce bleeding from an injury.

Vitamin K is a fat-soluble vitamin occurring in two forms for human consumption:

- Vitamin K1 (phylloquinone)
- Vitamin K2 (menaquinone).

Foods high in Vitamin K1 are:

- Leafy greens
- Broccoli

- Iceberg lettuce
- Oils such as soybean and canola oil.

Foods high in Vitamin K2 are:

- Full-fat dairy products
- Pork
- Poultry
- Fermented foods.

Since it is fairly easy to meet Vitamin K needs, deficiency is rare. Your doctor may recommend a vitamin K supplement if you have a condition that causes excessive bleeding or prevents proper vitamin K absorption.

If you have gallbladder or biliary disease, cystic fibrosis, celiac disease, or Crohn's disease, or take antibiotics for long periods of time, you may benefit from a vitamin K supplement. You should make this decision in consultation with your healthcare provider.

If you take blood thinners such as warfarin, you should talk with your healthcare provider before taking vitamin K supplements or increasing your intake of foods with vitamin K. If you are taking blood-thinning drugs, you should avoid extra vitamin K because it can reverse the effects of these drugs.

Calcium

Your calcium needs increase as you age, especially postmenopause. Again, please discuss your best choice with your healthcare provider. Our recommended intake is 1200 mg–2000 mg. Dairy products contain the highest amount of calcium in our food supply and have the highest absorption rate. However, to meet your daily calcium needs, you would need to include 3–4 servings of dairy products daily.

Calcium plays an essential role in maintaining our muscle and bone health. Typically, the amount that you need is higher than you may be able to include in your diet, so calcium supplements are typically recommended. Supplements are available in the form of calcium carbonate and calcium citrate. Calcium citrate is more easily absorbed if you have less acid in your stomach (which is common as we age). Your absorption is increased if you take 500 mg at a time rather than 1000 mg.

Magnesium

Magnesium is an important mineral that many are deficient in, especially as we get older. You may:

- Absorb less from your food due to aging or the chronic use of some medications, such as diuretics and proton pump inhibitors
- Excrete more magnesium in your urine as you age
- Consume less in your diet than you need
- Or a combination of all of the above.

Chronic magnesium insufficiency has been linked to inflammatory markers. Not having enough of this essential mineral has been linked to several health concerns, such as sleep disorders, impaired cognition, cardiovascular disease, stroke, type 2 diabetes, asthma, and depression.

Significant sources of magnesium in your diet are:

- Nuts and seeds
- Whole grains and beans
- Green and leafy vegetables
- Milk and yogurt
- Cocoa
- Fortified foods.

If these foods are not common in your diet, you may want to consider taking a dietary supplement.

Special consideration

When writing this book, there was little discussion of the special nutritional needs for those taking GLP-1 medications. I have several clients who are using these medications to manage their Type II diabetes while continuing to work on their recovery from eating disorders. I am paying close attention to possible malabsorption, deficiencies, and their unique nutritional needs in light of their decreased appetite and intake. At this point, I do not have any data to support particular dietary recommendations. I predict there will be attention to this topic in the future. At least, I hope there will be!

As we close this chapter, if you've been a dieter, following food rules have provided you with guard rails for your food choices. This chapter encourages you to remove the guard rails and turn toward your own body's wisdom, and instincts to nourish yourself. I've also included several general recommendations to support you in this process.

Overall, I hope this chapter supports nourishing you so that you live comfortably, confidently, and unapologetically in your midlife+ body. My vision is for your eating habits and preferences to help you prioritize your energy and well-being so that you can age how you would like. Now that you've gotten perspective on nourishment, let's turn our attention to movement.

7

Reclaiming playful movement

"A lot of what we've been taught about fitness is actually diet culture wrapped in spandex."

Shannon Palus

In Chapter 3, we discussed the damages you may have experienced at the hands of diet and anti-aging culture and how "diet and exercise" are interwoven in your perception and experience. This chapter picks up that discussion to support you in healing the damage done. Reminder: Many have experienced harmful shaming experiences associated with physical activity and exercise, so I use the word movement when referring to physical activity and exercise as much as possible to decrease the likelihood that you will feel triggered by these terms.

Let's begin this mending process with questions and journal prompts that help you become more aware of your relationship with movement. We can't change what we are not aware of, right?

Begin by connecting with your body, as described in previous chapters, and make yourself as comfortable as possible. Grab your journal and respond to these questions:

- If you were granted a day to do precisely as you wished, would your day include time to play? Would you go for a swim, ride a bike, dance or stretch yourself out on a field of grass, climb a hill to see a little further, or play a game of whatever sport you loved to play at some point in your life?

- What movement would interest you if you lived in a world free of concern about your body's size, shape, or composition?
- How does dropping all of the "shoulds" about moving your body alter your interest in movement, or does it?
- Are you on and off "exercise programs" just as you are on and off diets and food rules?
- Do you engage in movement to somehow compensate or punish yourself for eating?
- Do you feel you need to earn eating food by moving your body?
- Is movement a way to do "damage control" after eating food during a special occasion, such as a holiday or vacation, that you feel guilty or concerned about?
- As you ponder your response to these questions, are you noticing evidence that diet or anti-aging messages contaminated your relationship with movement?
- If so, are there feelings associated with this insight?
- How did you play as a kid? How do these memories feel in your body?
- Are you interested in returning to this kind of playing again, if you are able?
- Does your age affect how you feel about moving your body?
- Do you think your age makes you afraid to participate in any particular type of movement? If so, write more about this experience.
- Do changes in your body alter your ability to engage in any particular activity? If so, write more about this experience.
- Does your age increase your motivation to move your body?
- Is there anything else that complicates your relationship with movement?

As an aspect of your relationship with your body, your relationship with movement is likely complicated. This chapter is dedicated to understanding this complex relationship and beginning the mending process.

Positives of moving your body in midlife+

First, let's acknowledge the positives of movement. Research strongly correlates movement with:

- Joy and pleasure
- Potential for social connection
- Improved cognition and potentially slowing cognitive decline
- Slowing the loss of muscle mass, which decreases the risk of falling
- Protection of bone mass
- Improved sleep
- Improved mood
- Management of stress and anxiety
- Potential for nervous system regulation
- Improved metabolism due to support of muscle mass
- Supports management of blood sugar
- Supports management of blood lipids
- Supports management of blood pressure
- Improved balance, which decreases the risk of falling
- Eases pain from osteoarthritis and muscle tightness
- May boost immunity
- Opportunity for body connection and embodiment.

In his book *Keep Sharp*, Dr. Sanay Gupta praises the benefits of movement as "the single most important thing for brain function and mitigating disease." His recommendations align with the CDC's: be moderately active for at least 150 minutes a week—the equivalent of half an hour on five days or 50 minutes on three days. Alternating among varying speed, intensity, and effort levels with various activities is recommended. Including a couple of days of strength training in your exercise boosts your muscle, bone mass, and brain health.

Notably, all of the above benefits exist without a connection to changes in your body size or shape!

The harm of fitness culture

Diet and fitness culture have conflated moving your body with controlling your body size and shape. As a result, you need to clarify the many ways moving your body supports your well-being with absolutely zero change in your weight.

We humans have an innate need and desire to move our bodies. However, we often forget that we are animals. For example, when you observe animals, you see them get up and stretch their bodies after a nap. With some exceptions due to injury or illness, moving and stretching our bodies usually feels quite good.

At the same time, if you've ever been caught up in diet/fitness or anti-aging culture messages, experienced trauma at the hands of fitness culture or had an eating disorder, you likely lost your connection to your body's innate interest in movement.

I want to make this clear: You are not required to move your body to belong or to be loved. Movement is your choice. Approaching movement with a complete sense of agency supports your mending. Embedded within the conversation of agency, we must consider your capacity and your body's abilities.

Ableism

Before proceeding, we need to acknowledge the presence of ableism in diet/wellness and anti-aging/longevity culture. Both tend to exclude those with marginalized identities, including people with disabilities.

Every one of us will likely experience not being able to engage in movement as we would like at some point in the present or future. For most of us, aging will bring some form of disability if it hasn't already. We need to do a much better job of creating accessible and inclusive movement spaces. I've listed accessible movement resources I am aware of in the Resources section.

In addition to creating more inclusive and accessible movement spaces, several strategies would help to combat ableism as we age:

Strategy	Description
Inclusive movement programs	Develop and promote movement programs accessible for all body sizes and abilities.
Accessible facilities/spaces	Ensure movement facilities are accessible to all, including ramps, elevators, adaptive equipment, and clear signage. Create inclusive spaces where everyone feels welcome and supported.
Representation	Increase representation of bodies of all sizes, ages, races, gender identities, and abilities in movement media, marketing, and leadership roles.
Education and training	Provide education and training for movement professionals on creating inclusive environments and working with clients of all sizes and abilities.
Shift the narrative	Promote a broader definition of fitness that values movement for its benefits, enjoyment, and social connections rather than focusing on appearance, weight loss, or performance metrics. Emphasize that fitness is for every body, regardless of size, age, or ability.
Empowerment and advocacy	Encourage everyone to advocate for their needs within the movement community. Support creating opportunities for sharing lived experiences to encourage empathy and empowerment.

Ableism, anti-fat bias, weight stigma, sexism, transphobia, racism, homophobia, and ageism in fitness, yoga, and wellness spaces prohibit feeling safe, a sense of belonging, and enjoying movement for many. By promoting inclusive practices, increasing accessibility, and challenging negative stereotypes, the movement community can create a more welcoming and supportive environment for everyone. Embracing diversity in bodies and abilities emphasizes that fitness and health do not have a look!

You cannot know someone's health status or fitness capacity by looking at them. But you would never know this by following fitness trends and influencers. Feeling like your body is capable is challenging when you see bodies aligning with the ideal of thin, fit, young, white, able, cis-gendered, and beautiful dominating the movement influencer spaces.

Protecting yourself from harmful fitness influencers

Most fitness influencers on social media misrepresent the truth and may have a disordered relationship with their bodies, eating, and movement. Remember, they post to sell you something, whether that's a supplement, equipment, a program or aspirational lifestyle. They have their own biases on display. While I can empathize with their struggle, I take issue with the use of social media platforms to spread harmful, oppressive messages about bodies. So, how can you protect yourself?

- *Curate your feed*: Follow inclusive influencers who promote body diversity accessible movement and realistic goals. It is even more critical to unfollow accounts that make you doubt or judge yourself. Be picky! See Resources for recommended accounts. **Only follow accounts that leave you feeling supported and encouraged in the body you are in now.**
- *Limit your exposure*: Limit your exposure to social media. Research has established its negative effect on body image.
- *Carefully find support*: Instead of using social media as your source of guidance, carefully seek certified movement professionals to create an individualized program to meet your goals. It's a good idea to interview them to clarify your goals and set protective boundaries, like "no diet advice, no weight goals." You may also want to limit your exposure to being measured. You are the customer! See the Resources section for online sources.

- *Focus on your process*: Focus on your process and set accessible and sustainable individualized goals. Celebrate your wins along the way—there are no small wins!
- *Consumer be-aware*: Be discerning of the content you consume. Assess the credibility of the advice. Be-aware that some content may be sponsored and potentially biased.
- Remember, finding movement that brings playful enjoyment and pleasure into your life is a goal!

Sometimes, it helps to step away from fitness culture and return when you feel more comfortable and less vulnerable to the false promises and body criticism commonly found there. Unfollow all fitness accounts to take a break from being exposed to this content and images. And, when you're ready, slowly add accounts that support your mending process.

You may experience some resistance when you return to movement. How do you know you are experiencing exercise resistance (a part of you may be calling yourself lazy)?

Let's talk about a client whose experience with movement represents this common experience.

Mary Jane's story

Mary Jane was a 51-year-old woman, recently diagnosed with adult ADHD. Growing up, she didn't worry about her eating or movement and mainly felt comfortable with her body (as much as our culture allows). She transformed her life in her early 40s, shifting careers and heading back to school for a graduate degree. During grad school, though, she went through a divorce and gained some weight. She was also perimenopausal during this time.

A friend joined the women's triathlon and invited Mary Jane to join her there. Mary Jane accepted her invitation with excitement. Her children were teenagers and required less of her time with shared custody, and she was newly single, so she enjoyed the community and new friendships she made in the program. She began a demanding running, swimming, and biking schedule.

When she got together with her new friends, they frequently also talked about their diets. Curious, Mary Jane committed to

30 days of restrictive eating rules for a program popular amongst her new community. She began "clean" eating. Her body changed significantly due to this extreme increase in her activity level, and she completed the triathlon.

Then, after graduation, Mary Jane moved to another city for a new job. She no longer had the movement community she enjoyed and could not find a replacement in her new city. She missed many things about her previous life. Her perimenopausal symptoms became more intense as she approached menopause.

Still, she was happy with her new job and wanted to make a good impression, so she worked 50–60-hour weeks as a newbie in her field. However, her ADHD medication, which helped her focus and manage her time, also made her forget meals. When she signed off for the day, she felt intensely hungry. She now found herself eating past fullness in the evenings.

And then the pandemic hit. She started working from home and rarely went out. Isolated and alone, she could not sustain the rigid food rules of her previous eating plan. She found herself eating the foods she had been depriving herself of and sometimes binge eating. She experienced a new job, a new city, menopause, and the COVID-19 pandemic all within one year. Her body changed significantly once again.

She realized that she was depressed and was developing disordered eating patterns and decided to seek treatment with me. Together, we first addressed the straightforward issue of not eating enough during the day. We set up several quick, easy, and satisfying meals and snacks that met her needs. Then, we worked on mind-body practices to regulate her nervous system at the end of her work day. In the evenings, she resumed art projects she enjoyed. As COVID restrictions lifted, she started socializing after work. Her relationship with her food and eating were resolving with her significant efforts over time.

However, Mary Jane was very resistant to returning to any movement. She was not interested in returning to the intense program she had previously been involved in. She understood she was stuck in the "nothing" part of her all-or-nothing thinking about movement. The thought of trying small steps or something more comfortable or moderate did not feel like "enough to count" to Mary Jane. She did not realize it, but her perception of her previous experience with movement was very caught up in her experiencing significant changes in her body. Like it or not, she still wanted that, which is understandable!

Exercise resistance makes sense

Feeling resistant to returning to movement can be challenging and is a common aspect of the mending process. If you're trying to break up with diet and anti-aging culture, which includes fitness culture, it can be confusing when you decide to return to moving your body. Remember, your experiences with restriction and food rules were likely unpleasant; some would say traumatizing. Therefore, anything associated with previous periods of engaging with diet/wellness culture has an undesirable connotation.

Another source of resistance may be rooted in body grief. You may also be experiencing changes in your body and performance that affect your interest in participating. The "all or nothing" thinking of fitness and diet culture may have you clinging to the expectations of your younger body and performance. Therefore, you may want to resist movement to avoid experiencing your body performing differently.

Many of my clients tell stories of being disappointed that they are slower on the tennis court or when they run, making it hard for them to feel interested in continuing to engage. The potential for aches and pains, surgeries, and illnesses that change your body increases as you age, and body grief is associated with these body changes.

Take your time and be gentle with yourself. When you are ready, acknowledge the body changes you are experiencing. Allow yourself to feel the feelings associated with the ways your body moves and feels differently. I know that is easier said than done. You may even feel like your body is betraying you. These body changes may bring up feelings of loss and grief. Over time, you can accept these changes. Acceptance allows you to adapt so you can move on when you are ready.

A gentle reminder: The feeling that your body is betraying you as it changes often stems from the cultural belief that your body should stay the same and conform to a narrow ideal of a 'good body'. But your body isn't failing you—it's adapting, and evolving. Your body is doing a good job. When you can recognize that, it becomes easier to accept your body as it is and move forward with more ease and self-compassion.

When resistance is protective

Resisting an experience that once harmed you or brings up uncomfortable feelings is *protective*.

It is likely that your resistance is below your conscious awareness and goes unnamed. You may feel like you are lazy or lack willpower and discipline when, in fact, a part of you is looking out for you and has your best interest at heart!

Your fitness achievements or being an exercise enthusiast may have been part of your identity. You may have received so much affirmation for this part of your life that it dominated your identity. After receiving high praise for pushing yourself hard in the past, it can be complicated to be gentle with yourself and how you move your body.

Diet and fitness culture often encourages us to view moving our bodies through an "all or nothing" lens. If you no longer want to push yourself and excel by doing it all, you may feel that the alternative is doing nothing. It's challenging to find a middle ground and do "some" and let that be enough.

I hope that when you realize how hard you have been on yourself and how much you pushed yourself in the past, and the fact that a wise part of you doesn't want you to go through that again, this allows you to feel compassion for yourself. Can you feel grateful for that protective part of you? Thankfully, a part of you no longer wants you to suffer which is a sign you are healing.

Journal prompts

If you find returning to movement after a break or body change challenging, these prompts are for you. I encourage you to pause, give yourself the time and attention for a body check-in, practice, and pull out your journal to respond to these prompts.

- Do you feel uncomfortable or irritated when others talk about their exercise program or when you receive a recommendation to move your body? Describe your experience with special attention and curiosity about how this experience and your feelings show up as sensations in your body.
- Do you want to ditch your movement program when you see you are not losing weight or your body is changing the way you wanted? Describe emotions related to this desire to drop it. Are you feeling disappointed? Are you feeling angry? Are you feeling frustrated? Are you feeling sad? Are you feeling confused? Are you feeling a mix of some of these emotions or something different? Describe your experience with special attention to and curiosity about how these feelings show up as sensations in your body.
- Do you want to ditch your movement program when you see you are not performing like you once did? Describe emotions related to this desire to drop it. Are you feeling disappointed? Are you feeling angry? Are you feeling frustrated? Are you feeling sad? Are you feeling confused? Are you feeling a mix of some of these emotions or something different? Describe your experience with special attention and curiosity about how these feelings show up as sensations in your body.
- Do you feel guilt or shame when others discuss their movement or when you receive a recommendation to move your body? Describe this experience with special attention to and curiosity about how these feelings show up as sensations in your body.
- Is there anything else you are experiencing related to feeling resistant to moving your body or a complication related to moving your body?

As you begin to soften your inner dialogue about why you feel resistant to movement, you realize you must look at moving your body differently. The missing piece in your previous relationship to movement is likely pleasure and joy. Movement doesn't have to be transactional (you doing the time so your body will change). Adding the element of enjoyment and playfulness can help you find your way back.

Self-compassion plays a significant role in successfully navigating this tricky terrain, but other strategies exist for moving through your exercise resistance.

- *Reframe movement as real self-care*: See movement as a form of caring for your body rather than a means to fix a problem. Focus on the immediate benefits, such as improved mood, regulated nervous system, release of tension, and even a clear mind.
- *Include movement that you enjoy*: Of all the things you can do to mend your relationship with movement, finding ways to move your body that you genuinely enjoy is essential. Dancing, hiking, swimming, or yoga are key to finding movement that is fun and rewarding.
- *Set accessible goals*: Set realistic and achievable goals. Start small and take small steps so that you experience progress over time. There is no place for perfection! Celebrate small wins (and sometimes that is listening to your body and taking a day off) to build body trust, respect, and confidence.
- *Find community*: Search for a supportive and non-judgmental movement environment, even if it is online. Consider saying "yes" to joining group activities, finding a movement buddy, or participating in online movement communities that offer accessible movement and promote an inclusive environment.
- *Challenge anti-aging and diet culture narratives*: Actively dismantle anti-aging and diet culture narratives that tie movement to appearing young, losing weight, or your body's appearance. Focus on the fact that your age, body size, or appearance do not define your well-being.

Is more better? Exercise addiction in midlife+

Many of my clients describe feeling comfortable with a way of caring for themselves that kept their bodies in a particular "shape" and then suddenly, in midlife, finding their habits were no longer "working" to maintain the shape or size they were accustomed to. They increased their exercise duration, frequency, or intensity to control their changing bodies and soon slipped into excessive exercise that spiraled out of balance.

Margo Maine, Ph.D., and Joe Kelly, authors of *Pursuing Perfection: Eating Disorders, Body Myths, and Women at Midlife and Beyond*, included a list of aspects to ask yourself to determine if your relationship with exercise is healthy or excessive:

- I judge a day as good or bad based on how much I exercise.
- I base my self-worth on how much I exercise.
- I never take a break from exercise, no matter how I feel or how inconvenient it is.
- I exercise even though I am injured.
- I arrange work and social obligations around exercise.
- I cancel family or social engagements to exercise.
- I become angry, anxious, or agitated when something interferes with my exercise.
- I know others are worried about how much I exercise, but I don't listen to them.
- I always have to do more (laps, miles, weights) and rarely feel satisfied with my progress.
- I count how many calories I burn while exercising.
- I exercise to compensate for eating past the point of fullness.

Sometimes, your relationship with movement is complicated by its role in managing your emotions. Consider whether movement is your only way to cope with emotional discomfort or to regulate your nervous system. When movement is your *only* way to help yourself feel better, you risk abusing it. We'll get into additional practices to expand your options for regulating your nervous system in the next chapter.

When movement is entangled with anti-aging and diet culture rhetoric, and you are using movement to control your appearance or body size, this leaves you vulnerable to creating more dependence and overuse of movement, especially in midlife and beyond when you are experiencing body changes that feel out of your control.

From obligation to invitation: A new way to move

- *Cultivate a more balanced approach:* Include rest days and mix up the types of movement you enjoy. Remember that recovery following movement and rest are crucial to a healthy relationship with moving your body.
- *Practice body connection and respect:* Consider if movement in your life supports your whole-person well-being. You benefit from approaching movement with an attitude of moderation rather than the all-or-nothing way of thinking about movement you may have learned. See movement as an opportunity to connect with your body, listening to your body's feedback while respecting the need for rest and recovery periods.
- *Shift the focus away from weight management and muscle gain:* To develop a balanced and healthy relationship with movement, focus on its intrinsic benefits, such as improved mood, better sleep, enjoyment, and overall well-being, rather than external rewards like weight management or muscle gain.
- *Challenge anti-aging and diet culture rhetoric:* Actively commit to dismantling the narratives promoted by anti-aging and diet culture that equate excessive movement with moral virtue and ignore and override your body's wise requests for moderation and rest. *Remember: Bodies of all sizes, abilities, and sizes are worthy!*
- *Address underlying issues:* Becoming more curious about your relationship with movement may uncover concerns with perfectionism, obsessive thoughts, exercise compulsions, or an over-reliance on movement to manage anxiety and mood.
- *Find supportive connections and communities:* You may need to seek more support to address these underlying issues. You don't

have to do this alone! Find and join in supportive communities associated with movement where all bodies are welcome and include diverse bodies along with a healthy, balanced approach to movement. This can help you feel less isolated and more supported as you mend your relationship with movement.

The risks of overdoing it

There is a point where too much of a good thing can create more harm. In addition to the potential imbalance in your relationship with your body, eating, energy, relationships, and time, there is the potential for overuse injuries.

Overdoing it with exercise can increase your risk of muscle, joint, and bone injuries, especially if you've been diagnosed with osteoporosis or arthritis. Common injuries include overuse injuries, stress fractures, rotator cuff tears, and meniscus tears.

A study (Schnohr et al., 2015) tracked the health of 1,098 healthy joggers and 3,950 healthy non-joggers over 12 years from 2014. Light and moderate joggers (a speed of around 5 mph and no more than three times a week or for 2.5 hours in total) had lower mortality than otherwise healthy non-joggers. However, strenuous joggers (who ran at speeds higher than 7 mph or more than four hours a week) tended to die at a higher rate than light and moderate joggers and at a similar rate to healthy non-joggers! The link remained when factors such as age, sex, the history of heart disease or diabetes, smoking, and the levels of alcohol consumed were taken into consideration.

The most compelling conclusion of this study is that exercise's effects are horseshoe-shaped. Beyond a certain point, physical activity stops enhancing health and may start harming it. Striking a balance or a middle ground in your relationship with movement supports your well-being on multiple levels.

Addressing over-exercise involves recognizing the complex mix of body image, ageism, and diet culture, along with contributing psychological and social factors. What protects you from the risks of exercise addiction and supports a more balanced approach to movement?

- Cultivating a more embodied approach
- Working toward a flexible mindset
- Challenging anti-aging and diet culture rhetoric
- Finding a supportive and inclusive community.

Reclaiming playful movement

I've heard countless stories from my clients who were initially very motivated to start a movement program but soon experienced the new program as joyless drudgery, leading them to drop out. Sound familiar? From this experience, you might believe that you are too lazy, not committed or disciplined enough, or do not have the time or energy. Moving your body becomes "working out," painful, and something you "have to" do. The more you connect movement with changes in your body size or muscle building, the more likely you will feel frustrated if you do not see these changes immediately. You may wonder, "What's the point?" and give up.

It's no surprise that the majority of people who begin a movement program only continue it for a short time. According to the CDC (2022), as of 2020, 25.3 percent of Americans met the recommended guidelines for activity, which was at least 150 minutes per week of moderate-intensity aerobic physical activity or 75 minutes per week of vigorous-intensity aerobic physical activity, or an equivalent combination and muscle-strengthening activities on at least 2 days per week.

The thing is, playing and *enjoying your body* as you move is your birthright!

"Exercise" is something you've been told you "should" do in a particular way, for a specific amount of time, a certain number of days to get "results" by anti-aging and diet culture. This dogmatic messaging fractured your relationship with movement. You may have even experienced trauma and body shame related to this. So now, how can this fracture be mended?

You had an innate desire to move your body, but anti-aging and diet culture have robbed you of this. You need to return to your sense of agency and reclaim movement as a choice, a part of your life that can bring you joy and pleasure that you look forward to. You are in charge and can do as you please with your body, within your ability and interest.

From this perspective, you will be much more successful in creating a relationship with moving your body that you see as something you "get to do" and are likely to want to do again tomorrow if you:

- Reframe your movement as a form of play
- See movement as a source of pleasure
- Experience movement as another way to get to know yourself. Be curious about your body, and see movement as an opportunity to discover what moving is like
- Focus on movement as care and nurturance
- See movement as a way to connect with your body or practice embodiment
- Focus on movement as another potential source of social connection
- Notice potential positive side effects, such as:
  - A regulated nervous system
  - An energy boosts
  - Clear-headedness (less brain fog)
  - Potentially improved a sense of self-mastery.

I spoke with my colleague David Wilson to hear his take on the experience of moving our bodies in midlife and beyond.

Notes from an expert

David Wilson (@oldcoolmoves) is a movement educator, anti-ageism advocate, and speaker:

> As you age, your body inevitably evolves and changes. Your movement practice needs to meet you where you are, rather than in some mythical past or in the land of wishful thinking. You need to be more connected and curious about your body so that you can adjust your movement practice to the goals and the body you have now.
>
> Pay attention to how you're moving and how you're not moving. Our bodies are wise and wired for efficiency. For example, your body naturally rounds forward when sitting and working with your hands or reading. Over time, your muscles adjust to make finding and staying in this position easier. Certain muscles lengthen, and others shorten so that sitting in a rounded position uses less energy and requires less effort. The problem? It becomes difficult to restore a more neutral and elongated posture unless you regularly do things to counteract forward rounding.
>
> How you don't move influences how you can move. We get good at what we practice, but only those things. For example, walking is terrific and has many merits. However, it doesn't help you reach for a heavy pot in your cupboard, get up and down from the floor, or confidently leap out of the way of an oncoming skateboarder. So, when creating your movement practice, find a variety of movements that encourage the development of strength, coordination, flexibility, balance, and stability in all sorts of ways.
>
> The ultimate goal is to create a movement practice that supports how you want to be able to move in the world and that encourages you to move again tomorrow, avoiding pain and minimizing the risk of injury while inviting playfulness, delight, and pleasure.

I wonder if David's attitude were more common in wellness and fitness whether more of us would see movement as more accessible and would be moving our bodies more consistently!

Mary Jane's story continued

At the beginning of our work on Mary Jane's resistance to moving her body, she needed to give herself full and complete *permission not to move her body*. She acknowledged that pushing herself and feeling that she "should" move her body were not working. She had to practice, knowing she had permission to never exercise again, and she breathed a sigh of relief at that!

A few months into our work together, she felt more connected to her body and realized she wanted to stretch after sitting or sleeping. As a cat owner, this made her smile. In the spring, she became interested in gardening, which required various types of significant movement. She started seeing this as going outside to play.

With this new, active hobby that she genuinely enjoyed, Mary Jane became curious about other play options and began having little dance parties with herself in the kitchen at the end of her workday.

Eventually, she started wanting to go for weekend hikes with friends and her kids. Soon, she realized that she was doing various activities, some requiring strength, like gardening, and others challenging her cardio capacity, like hiking and dancing.

There were some rough spots, too. When she saw her healthcare provider for her annual complete physical exam, he mentioned being concerned about her BMI and weight. He asked if she had a "sedentary lifestyle" and if she would be interested in being referred to the medical center's "weight management program."

Mary Jane froze. Stunned and upset, the words got stuck in her throat. The flood of body shame overrode every argument in favor of her health. She could not advocate for herself even though she engaged in a lot of movement. (By the way, her blood pressure and all of her labs were "within normal limits.")

After this stigmatizing experience, Mary Jane stopped moving her body for a few weeks. She felt somewhat defeated and that her current movement was not "enough."

She processed this with her therapist, and I reminded her that movement was not about managing her weight. We created a list of the benefits she was experiencing, focusing more on her improved mood, feeling much less anxious, and sheer enjoyment. Soon after, she was able to re-engage with her movement favorites.

She even bought a bike and joined a biking club, which offered her a supportive community like she had before she moved. She talked about how much fun she was having. Mary Jane developed the identity of a woman who moves and plays, in addition to her efforts to nourish herself well and feel more confident in her body. She then graduated from my care, celebrating that she thought she had mended the fracture in her relationship with movement.

Journal prompts

Before you proceed, please take the time to make yourself comfortable and check in with your body. Arrive in your body, connecting with where your body meets a surface, and allow yourself to feel held and supported by the earth. Scan your body for places that feel tight and try to soften there. Notice where you feel your breath if that is comfortable for you, and settle into a connection with your body.

Now, respond to these inquiries in your journal:

- What would invite you to look forward to moving your body?
- Can you imagine joyful movement in your own life?
- Consider activities that you might enjoy doing for fun.
- Next time you are around kiddos, observe how they are having fun. What is the difference between what they're doing and what you and other adults do when engaging in movement?
- Imagine what you might do if you simply enjoyed moving your body.
- Begin by exploring the question: Exactly what excites you and prompts the question, "What do I get to do today?"

Just to give you some ideas, what about:

- Throwing a frisbee
- Jumping rope
- Trying a new online yoga class
- Meeting a friend for walking and talking
- Turning on some tunes and dancing while cooking dinner
- Signing up for a pickleball class

- Going for a swim
- Making love
- Walking the dog in a park across town
- Raking the leaves
- Asking the grandkids or neighborhood kids to play catch
- Signing up to rent a canoe or kayak at the lake.

Ask one of your beloveds to join the brainstorming and make your own list. Maybe even post it somewhere in sight so you don't drop the ball (see what I did there?).

Don't overdo it! Take it slow and stay curious about what you enjoy and what makes you feel good. As David Wilson advises, engage in a movement so that you "want to do it again tomorrow"! David's programs are listed in the Resources. He is exceptionally talented at making movement playful.

Movement that aligns with your values

David explained to me that there is some truth to the fact that as you become fit, you continually need to challenge your body to continue to achieve higher levels of fitness.

My question is, to what end? No shade if this is what you are after. Remember the long and data-supported list of benefits to movement, especially in this chapter of your life. I fully support you moving your body in whatever way you please, but you should feel like it is your choice and so you don't feel oppressed or manipulated.

For me personally, I value having a sharp mind so long as I can and enough energy and capacity for adventures. Movement that supports me in living these values and makes me feel alive interests me. More than anything, I ask myself: *Does this support me in feeling intimate with my experience?*

I am interested in movement that invites me to connect with my body as I move. Movement that disconnects me from my body and my experience does not interest me. Therefore, I prefer something other than gadgets and machines with numbers to motivate me to participate in movement. These interrupt or take me out of my experience.

Yoga, playing with my grandkids, dancing, hiking, kayaking, and biking outdoors all stimulate my interest, as do learning new ways of movement. Being able to be outdoors is a bonus!

You must clarify your values to find what interests you and motivates you from your heart; in other words, you must be intrinsically motivated. You know what I'm going to say, right?

You are the expert of you!

Embodied movement

You may have followed teachers, influencers, and guidelines, looked for outcomes, and checked devices for so long that you've forgotten to become curious about how moving your body feels to you.

You may have lost the thread of experiencing pleasure that comes with playfully moving your body. I love these wise words from my interview with Niamh Daly:

Notes from an expert

Niamh Daly (@yinstinctyoga), yoga teacher and author of *Yoga for Menopause and Beyond*:

> I want to help people feel more connected and comfortable in their bodies by focusing on functional and playful movement. Something missing in the Wellness and Fitness world's approach to movement is helping people travel the final decades of their lives aware of and enjoying the tickles of pleasure experienced when they move their bodies.

Reconnecting with the experience of noticing what your body feels like when you move will help you form a new relationship with movement. What happens when you stay curious about noticing "the tickles of pleasure experienced when you move your body" as Niamh says?

Pay attention to how it feels to move your body any amount while cultivating a more curious and playful attitude. The intention is to increase your connection to the sensations you experience when moving your body and, potentially, your awareness of joy in movement.

As a yoga student and teacher, I learned that the most subtle movement often creates the greatest opportunity to get to know your body. Let's do a little experiment.

Embodiment journal prompts/experiment

- Before you do anything, notice how you are holding your body in this moment. What gets your attention?
- What part of your body is touching a surface? How does that connection feel? Supportive? Uncomfortable? Uneasy or insufficient? Imposing or too much? Neutral? Does anything else come up for you when you notice your body meeting this surface?
- Check in with your appetite. Are you hungry? Satisfied? Craving? Full? Neutral?
- Notice the temperature of the air on your skin and your sense of your body's temperature. Are you a little chilly? Neutral? Too warm?
- Would you like to make any adjustments? If so, how did it feel to shift and move your body?

Move your body in a way you would call playful, which is entirely up to you! What anyone else may think about this is insignificant. You can move from a bed or chair or while leaning against the support of a wall or chair. Please follow your instincts and take care of yourself.

- Play music and move your body as the music invites you to move. You may want to play music to do any of the following:
  - o Hop, skip, and jump any amount your body feels safe doing.
  - o Stretch your arms up and your legs out any amount. Inhale as you stretch out and exhale as you release.
  - o Wiggle your fingers and toes, circle your ankles and wrists.
  - o Slowly swirl and twirl your body.
  - o Find or create water and move in any way that feels good.
  - o Take photographs of yourself making playful expressions with your face in a mirror.
  - o Roll around on a bed or the floor or ground outside if you are comfortable getting up and down from the floor or the ground.
  - o Play a game that you enjoy.
- When this experiment is complete, check in with yourself to see how you are feeling. Are there any echoes of this play in your body?
- Has anything shifted in your:
  - o Energy?
  - o Thoughts?
  - o Feelings or mood?
  - o Sensations of your body?
- Would you like more of this in your life? Or not?

Befriending your body as you move

As you shift away from oppressive anti-aging and fitness culture rules to reclaim movement, you are also befriending your body. The elements of this process include:

- Disentangling from external guidance and gadgets
- Practicing touching base with your body to inquire about what would feel good, what you have the energy for, and what you are in the mood for

- Moving so that you connect with your body's sensations and enjoyment
- Focusing on how your movements support your well-being
- Disentangling from rhetoric, mirrors, and gadgets focusing on your body's size and shape
- Nourishing and fueling your body's ability to engage in movement
- Moving and playing so you look forward to continuing to move and play
- Trying not to think of movement as a way to compensate or punish yourself for eating
- Being gentle and compassionate with yourself. It doesn't help to push yourself
- Giving yourself permission to take days off, slow down, and rest.

Reading this book may be your starting point for your mending process. The Resources section includes sources to support incorporating these elements more deeply into your life.

Now, let's discuss the importance of rest, sleep, and regulating your nervous system, which are equally as important as nourishment and movement for your well-being in midlife and beyond.

8

The embodied pause—the gifts of glimmers, rest, and sleep

"If you stay too busy to realize that your circumstances have changed, you don't notice that what you were running from is no longer chasing you. You won't realize that you have survived and can now move toward thriving."

Octavia F. Raheem, Rest Is Sacred

One of the most profound lessons I've learned, professionally and personally, is the healing nature of the embodied pause. By that I mean feeling, in real-time, the ground beneath my feet; enlivened by the elusive balance of effort and ease; and nourished by a forward fold that returns me to my center following a back bend. Each inhalation brings fresh, new energy with the oxygen I am breathing in, and each exhalation releases what is no longer helpful. I am reminded of the lessons of geese in flight—effort, effort, then glide.

This chapter's discussion of rest, sleep, and the restoration of your nervous system is an invitation to return to pause and return to your center after discussing the effort of mending your relationship with nourishment and movement.

Acknowledging that resting, sleeping well, and regulating our nervous systems may be the most significant true challenge we face in midlife and beyond. This chapter delves into the latest research findings supporting rest and sleep. We'll also explore the barriers and challenges we face when it comes to resting and getting a good night's sleep and discuss practices that support restorative rest and deep sleep in our lives.

In this chapter, we turn toward repairing the damage of diet culture and ageism. Let's begin with a quick recap of your nervous system, and how you can learn to regulate your nervous system, bringing a sense of embodiment and supporting your well-being.

Nervous system—a starting place

Your nervous system is a complicated and vast network of neurons whose primary role is to generate, modulate, and transmit information between your body's parts. It regulates vital bodily functions (cardiac function, breathing, digestion), sensations, and movements. Ultimately, your nervous system presides over everything that makes you human: your consciousness, thoughts, behaviors, and memories.

The vagus nerve is the longest cranial nerve and travels from your brainstem to various organs throughout your body, including your heart, lungs, and digestive tract. It plays a key role in regulating your heart rate, controlling muscle movements in your voice box, and managing various functions in your digestive tract. It's also involved in your body's relaxation response, helping reduce stress and promoting calmness. In recent years, research has focused on the role the vagus nerve can have in conditions like depression, anxiety, and inflammation.

You probably have experiences that illustrate the involvement of your vagus nerve in your response to stressful or traumatic events. Many years ago, I was in a car accident. I was very fortunate in that I was not seriously injured, and the only real symptom I had afterward, other than feeling shaken up and sore, was that I lost my voice, which surprised me. My healthcare provider called it a "stress response." My son was still an infant, and I was early in my career seeing patients and teaching at an academic medical center. That was 35 years ago, and I still wonder if I felt like I had too many responsibilities in my life to allow myself to slow down and feel how terrified I was, but my body manifested the trauma. The vagus nerve enervates the larynx or voice box. As Bessel van der Kolk, MD, renowned trauma researcher and psychiatrist says, "The body keeps the score."

In our modern lifestyle, many factors stress your nervous system and create dysregulation, and many of these stressors are heightened during midlife+. Trauma, chronic stress, genetic predisposition, environmental stress, systemic oppression, and hormonal changes in perimenopause and menopause contribute to nervous system dysregulation. I am reminded of these wise words from a a training session I participated in with Michael Stone and Molly Harris:

"What needs to be understood about trauma is that it's not the painful experiences we've had, it's the *impact* that those experiences have had on us. Because trauma increases stress and decreases trust, it takes a considerable physical and emotional toll and profoundly affects how we relate to each other.

We believe that it is our collective responsibility to find ways to understand, support, and create healing possibilities for ourselves and one another—as well as to examine and repair the systems, institutions, and inequities that create the conditions for trauma in the first place."

-Adapted from Michael Stone and Molly Boeder Harris

Nervous system dysregulation can feel like you are stuck in overdrive or hypervigilance, shut down, or numbed out.

Triggers and nervous system dysregulation

Triggers are people, places, things, or situations that make you feel unsafe or threatened. Triggers activate your sympathetic nervous system. Some examples of triggers include:

- Trying on clothes that fit your body differently
- Hearing people comment on the appearance of other people's bodies, or "aging"

- Seeing a pop-up ad or social media post that includes "before and after" pictures
- Seeing a photograph of yourself that jars or surprises you.

Sometimes, returning to a place or seeing people from a time when you experienced a great deal of dieting, over-exercising, or disordered eating we often hear can trigger dysregulation. Unfortunately, ageism is so common that ageist comments which can be triggering, "Aren't you too old to be doing that?"

At one point in my life, I was into mountain biking, and I wiped out on a challenging trail in the beautiful Great Smoky Mountains. I was left with some significant bruises but nothing more. But one of these bruises remained six months later, so I went to my primary care provider to have it checked out. She reacted with concern, saying that she wanted to rule out a soft-tissue sarcoma and referred me to an oncologist.

As I sat in the exam room waiting to see the oncologist, feeling very uneasy, the medical intern came in first to gather some information about me and my situation. When the attending physician arrived outside my door, I could hear his conversation with the medical intern, and I heard him exclaim, "What is she doing mountain biking at 45 anyway?!" Guess which part of this whole situation triggered me? I informed him that his patients could hear what he said at the exam room door, by the way.

Body image and dysregulation

In Chapter 4, we discussed feeling marginalized if your body does not "fit" in our youth and thin-obsessed culture; the longer you live, the more likely you are to experience body shame, weight stigma, chronic dieting, and eating disorders, which are experienced as trauma and contribute to the dysregulation of your nervous system. Depending on your internalized ageism and the ageism you encounter daily, growing older may also leave you feeling pushed to the margins, invisible or irrelevant.

Many of my clients report feeling less secure when they gain weight, become less able-bodied, and grow older. Unsurprisingly, these changes in your body contribute to your risk of feeling like you no longer belong and, therefore, becoming dysregulated occasionally or more frequently.

I want you to be able to recognize this and learn to regulate your nervous system. I also want to be clear that this is a systemic issue that I hope we can address by raising awareness of how we marginalize bodies and working to create a more inclusive culture. More about this in Chapter 10!

Nervous system dysregulation complicates your relationship with your body. This rupture makes it hard for you to notice your body's cues of hunger, satisfaction, and fullness or your desire to move and play. When dysregulated, you may seek regulation by over-exercising or not moving, not eating (being empty), only wanting to eat safe or familiar foods, or eating past fullness. Trauma and disordered eating patterns commonly co-occur. Mending your relationship with your body typically requires learning to regulate your nervous system.

Your window of tolerance

So, how do you know when your nervous system is regulated? The window of tolerance is a concept originally developed by Dr. Dan Siegel, MD, to describe the optimal zone of "arousal" for a person to function in everyday life. When you operate within this window, you are fully connecting with your body and receiving your body's cues.

Within your window of tolerance, you are centered, flexible, open, curious, present, emotionally regulated, and able to tolerate your life's stressors. You can pick up on your body's cues, and you have access to the part of your brain responsible for executive functioning and access to your wise self.

When you are "triggered" and outside your window of tolerance, you no longer have access to your executive functioning. You may revert to old, less functional thought and behavior patterns, affecting your eating, movement, and how you talk to yourself and care for your body.

The good news is that some practices help you expand your window of tolerance and regulate your nervous system. The goal is to be able to restore your regulation when you find yourself dysregulated.

Glimmers and regulating your nervous system

Glimmers, a term coined by trauma specialist Deb Dana, LCSW, are the moments in your day when you notice a sense of ease, connection, pleasure, and safety. These experiences support the regulation of your nervous system and help you feel grounded and connected to yourself and others. These moments offer a big payout: they bring you joy, happiness, peace, or gratitude, and fortunately they are simple and part of your everyday life.

Glimmers activate your parasympathetic nervous system, which supports your ability to "rest and digest." Some examples of glimmers include noticing the sun sparkling through the leaves, getting a warm hug from a beloved, feeling the warmth of a mug of tea in your hands, or basking in the warmth of the water on your back in the shower.

A resilient nervous system supports your optimal well-being at every age. Regulating yourself ensures that your body adapts to changes in your environment and maintains homeostasis or balance. This includes:

- Regulating your response to stressors
- Sleep regulation
- Appetite and digestion
- Mood management

- Focus and attention
- General functioning of all bodily systems.

Yes, your nervous system must be able to activate when there's a threat. You are brilliantly wired to protect yourself and survive. However, getting stuck in survival response or dysregulation does not serve you well. Your body is designed to re-regulate naturally. But as we discussed earlier, trauma affects your ability to regulate. If re-regulating does not feel like your strong suit, you may benefit from learning more self-regulating skills. Working with a therapist specializing in trauma and somatic practices may be helpful. You can develop an improved capacity to return to a state of calm, presence, and connection with practice.

There are various ways to engage your parasympathetic nervous system and self-regulate. This is a summary of accessible options. Please experiment and take what might work for you and leave the rest:

- Time in nature
- Slow, conscious movement such as restorative yoga, tai chi, or qigong
- Connection with your senses and noticing the sensations of your body
- Time with and the touch of loved ones or a pet
- Gentle movement such as a walk or a bike ride
- Listening to music or playing an instrument
- Creating art, doodling, or engaging in making crafts
- Laughing at a comedy show
- Watching a familiar or favorite show or music (the key here is familiar and comforting)
- Spiritual practice (this can be complex; if your practice induces shame and guilt, maybe not)
- Deep breathing, if that is comfortable for you, or tapping practices.

Sometimes, the repetitive motion of folding laundry, watering my garden, or the soothing experience of taking a bath regulates my nervous system, so it doesn't have to be complicated or novel! You are unique, so you may need to explore and see what works best for you. You may already know exactly what works best for you.

Both strengthening your ability to re-regulate your nervous system and preventing dysregulation, as best you can, will contribute to a more resilient nervous system and your well-being.

A sense of belonging and being seen by those around you provides a feeling of safety.

By combining the act of dismantling the internalized ageism and anti-fat bias you carry with protecting yourself from ageism and diet/wellness culture as much as possible (through boundary setting), you will decrease your dysregulation over time. This is a challenging endeavor! Developing awareness and taking small steps with these practices over time will make a big difference in your ability to find more peace of mind, body, and spirit. There is no need to rush yourself; take your time and be gentle with yourself. Expecting that you will do this perfectly, in a straight line, with no missteps on a timeline **contributes to your dysregulation.**

Learning to regulate your nervous system supports many aspects of your well-being and genuinely affects your sleep patterns, profoundly affecting your health in midlife and beyond. And vice versa. Providing your body with supportive care, like making space for rest, getting enough sleep, moving, and nourishing your body, all work together to improve your capacity for a resilient nervous system.

Body check-in and journal prompts

Now that you are more familiar with your nervous system, dysregulation, and the window of tolerance, let's focus on these concepts for your body check-in. For this practice, review the ideas listed above to engage your parasympathetic nervous system.

First, do what you need to do to arrive in your body at this moment. Perhaps create subtle movements, check in with your senses, notice where you are making contact with a surface, and allow yourself to feel held and supported by the earth beneath you. Scan your body for any places where you may be holding tension. Notice your breath and where you can feel it—no need to change it, simply notice.

Think of something relatively small that has upset you lately and caused you to feel dysregulated. When you remember this incident, scan your body for any sensations associated with your feelings and notice where you feel it. Can you bring yourself into your window of tolerance with some of the abovementioned ideas? Scan your body again and notice what may have shifted.

Journal prompts

Exploring how you've experienced nervous system dysregulation—and identifying what helps you return to your window of tolerance—can be profound.

Here are some journal prompts to guide your reflection:

- *Understanding your baseline*: Remember a time when you felt calm, safe, and grounded. What sensations do you notice in your body? What activities, environments, or people make you feel most at ease?
- *Noticing dysregulation*: Imagine a recent experience when you felt overwhelmed, anxious, or shut down. How did you experience this in your body (like nausea, heart palpitations)? What thoughts or stories were running through your mind?
- *Recognizing regulation practices*: What practices or tools might help you feel settled when stressed? Do you remember a time when you returned to a sense of calm after dysregulation? What helped bring you back?

Making space for rest

Due to the grind of feeling like we "should" be working on our bodies due to diet/wellness and anti-aging/longevity culture's constant focus on working on our body projects, we often overlook the importance of rest. The shifts and changes in our lives, relationships, and hormones make midlife and beyond a particularly stressful time. For most of us, rest was rarely modeled for us, so you may even feel like you don't know how. You may feel like being productive makes you worthy. You may feel lazy, guilty or unproductive if you take the time to rest. In fact, this couldn't be farther from the truth. It is counterintuitive, but sometimes, taking the time to rest requires much effort because we are pushing against learned beliefs.

"Grind culture has normalized pushing our bodies to the brink of destruction," Tricia Hersey writes in her essential book *Rest Is Resistance: A Manifesto*. "We are praised and rewarded for ignoring our body's need for rest, care, and repair."

Rest is freedom from activity or labor; it is a break from effort or movement to relax, refresh yourself, or recover strength. If you have ever trained for an athletic competition or event or worked with a personal trainer to enhance your fitness, you may have been advised to take rest days. Rest is part of the equation that includes movement and nourishment when building your body's capacity. The importance of rest extends beyond your body. Resting your brain offsets stress and overwhelm, preventing the increasingly common and very real phenomenon of "burnout."

My experiment with pausing

Let's begin with some context. As I write, I am in the midst of a presidential election. Three weeks ago, my region suffered the destruction of two back-to-back hurricanes, highlighting the stark reality of climate change. I am deeply concerned about the outcome of this election, our planet, and the people and land of Appalachia, so I have been glued to sources of information about all of this.

I started noticing signs that my nervous system was dysregulated. My sleep was noticeably restless. I was having a hard time focusing. I was beginning to feel hopeless. I was just so tired. Dealing with some resistance, I decided to practice what I preach.

1 I took a break from the news cycle, checking in only once daily to stay informed of the most essential information.
2 I became more consistent with my meditation practice.
3 I played with my grandkids and my pup.
4 I added dancing to my midday break.
5 I talked to my friends about how I was feeling.
6 I added some breathing exercises to manage hyperarousal.
7 I only watched shows that felt light to my spirit and made me laugh.
8 I wrote the word PAUSE on my inner left wrist to remind me to do just that.

I'm happy to report that I responded well to these changes. My sleep markedly improved, and I felt much less tense and had moments of levity—when I could follow these new guidelines I set for myself. But sometimes, I lapsed. I got seduced back into social media and sometimes did not take time for my meditation and breathing practices. When I dropped the thread of caring for myself, I also felt a decrease in my ability to be present and enjoy myself.

I am curious about my default impulse to lean toward working harder rather than giving myself a break. Can you relate? We've been taught to put our heads down and push through, but does that serve us? We know that chronic stress contributes to multiple mental and physical health issues over time.

We would benefit from learning a new way to respond when things are complex and we feel overwhelmed. Pause, give yourself a break, and rest first. Then, you can choose how to proceed from the more regulated and restored place you've created within yourself.

Rest is a power move

Rest is another delicious example of honoring your body's cues. Do you come up with more creative ideas or solutions to problems when you take a break from your effort, like when you take a shower or go for a stroll? Resting involves connecting to your present-moment experience—not worrying about the future or your past. In doing so, you support your ability to notice your body's cues and restore trust in your relationship with your body. Being in midlife and beyond is a brilliant time to learn to rest. I know, this can also be a time when you are feeling pressed to care for everyone else so it's not easy—that's why it's a power move!

By learning to rest, you are reassuring your body, specifically your nervous system, that you are safe. You can repair and rejuvenate within this sanctuary of safety you create for yourself. From this place of connection and access to your wise self, you can learn to relate to your body with more respect and care.

Clients tell me that when they deliberately pause at the choice points they pepper throughout their days, their effort to heal their relationships with eating, movement, and bodies have more momentum. Pausing creates the space to choose what, when, and how much you eat, move, and relate to your body with kindness and respect. While pausing, taking breaks, and resting have the potential to shift your process into gear, it is also challenging to allow yourself this softening. So, how can you learn to pause and rest if you are resistant?

Remember that your resistance is protective. A part of you learned and still believes you must keep working to be safe and seen as worthy, belonging, loved, or relevant. Because your busyness is protective, slowing down, pausing, and resting can feel vulnerable. Maybe when you take a break from busyness, that is when you notice uncomfortable thoughts and emotions. Can you be curious about your resistance to resting—with compassion, please?

What small shift could help you pause and breathe today?

Remember, we are all unique in what activities we find restful, and various situations may require different types of rest. If you've been sitting and focusing at your desk for long periods, you may take a break by moving your body, connecting with your breath and body sensations. Or, if you've been gardening for a while, you may need to rest quietly in a hammock with your eyes closed while you rest your ears on the sounds of the birds. Sometimes you only have a moment or two, so simply finding a way to look up at the sky and say a prayer, hum a tune, or say an affirmation can make all the difference. You have many options to experiment with.

The ultimate shift is in mindful connection to your present moment via the felt sense of your body.

Consider gathering any items you might use for your rest practice and keep them in one area of your home to invite yourself to take a break more consistently:

- Journal and pen
- Affirming/supportive book or cards (recommendations included in the Resources section at the back of the book)
- Pillows or bolsters
- Blankets
- Eye pillow
- Yoga mat
- Meditation cushion
- Musical instrument
- Art or craft supplies or coloring book/colored pencils

- Scented candle or essential oil
- A "Pause Playlist" on your music streaming service. (I made one on Spotify if you want to check it out! See the link in the resource section).

Pause and rest practices or rituals

I don't usually recommend committing to a daily practice, but committing to pause, take a break, and rest each day is an exception. You would benefit from daily practices that regulate your nervous system so that you can rest and sleep well. Here are a few options for varying lengths of time for you to play with. Check the Resources section for more.

Pause and rest practices and rituals

Morning rituals

- Take a 2–3-minute pause in the morning before you get hooked by your "shoulds" or your phone. When you open your eyes, place your hands on your heart and offer yourself some love and care with words of affirmation, gratitude, or a simple check-in with your body. My personal practice is to connect with my body by placing one hand on my heart and the other on my belly and ask myself, "What do I need to care for myself today?"
- Make time for a 5-minute pause as you drink your morning beverage and drop into connection with your senses—feel the warmth or coolness of the cup in your hands, breathe in the scents around you, let your ears rest on the sounds, savor the taste.
- Before you begin your day, pause for a moment and notice the sensation of your feet meeting the floor or where your body meets a surface. If you find it helpful, notice your breath. Allow yourself to scan your body to notice any places that may get your attention, and wonder how you might take action to offer your body a little more comfort as you begin your day. It may be as simple as stretching your neck, circling your shoulders, or wiggling your jaws.
- Create a 5–20-minute morning sitting or walking meditation practice.

- Make time for a 15–60-minute morning mindful movement practice, such as gentle or restorative yoga, tai chi, or qigong. You can find local or online options by conducting an online search.
- Savor your first meal of the day.
- Allow yourself a 15–30-minute expressive practice with art, music, or writing.
- Enjoy a 5–15-minute snuggle or romp with your pet!
- Enjoy a 5–30-minute snuggle or connection with your beloved.
- Enjoy your morning spiritual practice.

Mid-day break rituals

- 20–30-minute yoga nidra (my personal favorite!)
- 20–30-minute nap (or whatever amount of time leaves you restored and does not disrupt your sleep schedule).
- 15–30-minute mindful walk, bike, or swim.
- 5–30-minute conversation with your beloved.
- Your mid-day spiritual practice.

End-of-day rituals

- 20–60-minute restorative yoga practice.
- 15–60-minute creative practice that regulates your nervous system.
- 5–30-minute breath practice that regulates your nervous system.
- Savor bedtime tea while dropping into connection with your senses—feel the warmth of the cup in your hands, breathe in the scents around you, and let your ears rest on the sounds.
- 5–30-minute snuggle or conversation with your beloved.
- 5–30-minute snuggle with your pet.
- 30+ minute yoga nidra for sleep practice.
- 5–30-minute journaling to review your day, notice what you did well, notice what you will let go of for now and you can attend to later. Noteworthy, acknowledge what you did well helps to offset your negativity bias!
- 5–15-minute gratitude practice.
- 5–30-minute meditation practice.
- 30–60 minutes listening to calming or ambient music.
- Your end-of-day spiritual practice.

Cultivating practices that help you regulate your nervous system will also help you sleep well, so it's well worth your effort. A good night's sleep is elusive and golden in midlife and beyond!

How to make rituals and practices stick

If you find it challenging to stick with the practices and rituals you are trying, here are a few ideas to successfully integrate these new ideas into your life.

- Start with *small steps*. Large, sweeping changes are rarely sustainable.
- Experiment with *one new practice at a time*. When this starts to feel "automatic" and it is more comfortable, you can try your next practice.
- *Let your daily life be your reminder*. Your daily life has a rhythm, even when it feels chaotic. For example, you likely stop and nourish yourself 3–6 times each day. What if you try a grounding, self-compassion or body scan practice before you take your first bite?
- *Tracking* may help. Checking in with yourself each morning to plan when you will add your new ritual or practice and at the end of the day, noticing when you tried your new practice helps build it into your memory so that you are more likely to do it again and again. If tracking triggers diet culture, all-or-nothing thinking, or judgment, skip it for now.
- Expect to mess up, add your *self-compassion practice*, get curious about what's working and what is not, and begin again.
- Being *patient* with yourself may be the most critical skill of all.
- *Practice, practice, practice*. Nothing really changes without practicing.

I became an avid white-water kayaker when I was in my forties. I was divorced, and a single mom, and I needed something just for me. My instinct told me that I needed to try something new outside my comfort zone to restore my confidence and trust in myself and others. So, I joined a white-water club. To kayak white water, you must learn one critical skill: how to roll your kayak when your boat flips, and it will.

First, I took my boat to a pool with more experienced kayakers I trusted. I repeatedly turned my boat upside down, flipped myself right side up, and learned to roll my kayak. I practiced and practiced and practiced until I felt more comfortable. After I started feeling confident with my skill level, I took my boat to a lake, where, again with the support of others, I rolled and rolled until I was ready for a river. Of course, the rivers in the early days were gentle until I progressed and could roll my kayak in rapids. The trick is to practice so much that your body knows what to do (muscle memory) when your brain may be overwhelmed. Hanging upside down in a boat heading into rapids meant an overwhelmed brain for me! Eventually, I got the hang of it because my body knew what to do, and I trusted myself. Mission accomplished. Bonus, I made new friends and had the time of my life!

The ingredients to my success were:

- Small steps
- Loads of practice
- Support from people I trusted.

I would say the same about my self-compassion and somatic practices, and my yoga and meditation practices. I let my daily life remind me:

- When I am waiting for the kettle to boil I check in with myself, do a body scan, and offer myself compassion if needed (I usually need it!).
- When I brush my teeth, I either practice balancing on one foot or a mantra that I've been working with or both.
- When I go for a walk, I try to stay present to my body sensations or nature, looking for the glimmers, or both.

- When I have a natural interruption, like when my phone dings or I am at a stop light, I feel my feet or my seat, inviting me into connection with my body and check in with myself.
- When I drink a beverage, I allow the temperature of the mug or glass to remind me to check in with myself.
- When I am driving and someone cuts me off in traffic, I try to practice regulating my nervous system.

Of course, I don't do this perfectly! Life is messy! Sometimes, I forget all about these practices and then I remember and begin again. Most of these practices have taken me many years to develop. Please be patient with yourself.

Sleep and your well-being in midlife+

Sleep is crucial to health and well-being at every age, as it helps your body restore and repair itself. During sleep, your body produces hormones that aid tissue repair and growth. Sleep is also vital to the function of your immune system, protecting you from illness and disease; it is critical to maintaining your cognitive function, memory, and mood.

Health experts now believe sleep is "the foundation" of your well-being, especially in midlife and beyond.

What is a good night's sleep?

There is a common myth that we need less sleep as we age. According to the National Sleep Foundation (NSF, 2017) and Centers for Disease Control and Prevention (CDC), adults (18–65) require somewhere between 7–9 hours of sleep per night, and people aged 65 and older require around 7–8 hours. So basically, regardless of age, we function best as adults with around 8 hours of sleep, which does not change when we are older. As always, some outliers need as little as 6 hours and as much as 9 hours.

You and I both know we feel more rested some mornings than others. There is also a difference in the quality of our sleep. According to the CDC, sleep quality is as important as quantity. Poor-quality sleep contributes to brain fog, problems with memory, your capacity to learn new things, and overall daily functioning. Good quality sleep improves emotional regulation, immune function, blood sugar stability, and overall brain health and function.

Sleep experts agree on a few factors that impact the feeling of having had a good night's sleep, specifically fewer awakenings throughout the night, less time spent awake after initially falling asleep, and the electrical quality of your deep sleep.

Poor sleep quality leaves you feeling tired even though you technically got enough hours of sleep. Repeatedly waking up during the night and having sleep disorder symptoms are also indications of poor sleep quality. Addressing sleep disorders is essential to enhance the quality of your sleep and well-being.

According to the NSF, good quality sleep allows your body and brain to restore, supports optimal cardiac health, improves energy levels, and positively impacts mood. It supports your memory and cognitive function, enabling the brain to grow, reorganize, and form new neural pathways to support your ability to learn new information and form memories. Poor quality sleep can mean you have increased risks of mental distress, anxiety, depression, and irritability. It impairs clear thinking, memory formation, learning ability, and overall daily function. The quality of your sleep also influences blood sugar regulation.

The NSF also emphasizes the importance of sleep regularity, which is defined as the consistency of sleep–wake timing from day to day. A regular sleep routine supports your metabolic, cardiovascular, and inflammatory markers.

One of the NSF's most exciting findings was the concept of *chronotypes*, which are your body's natural preferences for wakefulness and sleep, influenced by your genetics and circadian rhythms. **Listening to and respecting your body's preferences improves your sleep quality, energy, and mood.** Chronotypes, such as being an early bird or a night owl, also influence your appetite, exercise, and body temperature, reflecting alertness and sleepiness at different times. I love it when science confirms what our bodies already know!

So now that we've established the importance of a good night's sleep, I know you know sleeping well is one of the ultimate challenges in midlife and beyond. There are some things you can do to get a good night's sleep.

A good night's sleep—easier said than done!

Hormonal changes, increased losses and stressors, body aches and pains, and increased anxiety often experienced in midlife and beyond all contribute to the elusive nature of a good night's sleep in this chapter of our lives. But there are strategies to improve your chances. Be patient with yourself and give these ideas some time to affect your body and brain before you call it.

Strategies for a good night's sleep

Here are some strategies sleep experts recommend for improving your sleep. As always, you are the expert of you, so take what works best for you and leave the rest! Feeling pressured about sleeping better defeats the purpose, so ease these ideas into your life.

Before bed

- Get sunlight during the day to help regulate your circadian rhythm and support your connection to your chronotype.
- Limit caffeine consumption, mainly after noon.
- Move your body during the day and limit strenuous movement close to your bedtime.
- Avoid alcohol consumption before bed, as it can disrupt your sleep later in the night.

Bedroom environment

- Keep your bedroom cool, dark, and quiet.
- The recommended temperature for optimal sleep is 68F / 20C degrees or less.
- If your bedroom is not sufficiently dark, consider using an eye mask or blackout curtains to create darkness.
- Keep a notepad and pen by your bed.
- If intrusive or ruminating thoughts keep you awake, dump them into your notepad. You can deal with these issues tomorrow and not at this very moment. Let them go with every exhale.

Right before bed

- Create a relaxing evening routine and bedtime ritual.
- Limit screen time.
- You may feel like you need to keep your phone within reach for safety purposes. But, as best you can, leave devices in another room to help you avoid using phones, tablets, or computers in bed.
- Orgasms or sexual activity at bedtime are encouraged if they help you relax.
- Yoga nidra for sleep is beneficial (see Resources for details).
- Practice imagining that you are bringing all the energy you give to the world, others, and projects and reclaiming your energy as your own. Turn your attention inward. This time is yours to rest and restore.

Set yourself up for success

- Address sleep concerns.
- If you suspect sleep apnea or other sleep disorders, consult your doctor for diagnosis and treatment. Don't put this off!
- Develop a consistent sleep schedule based on your body's preference.
- Go to bed and wake up close to the same time every day, even on weekends.

I know from experience that anxiety about not sleeping well can contribute to not sleeping well. If you have done all of your tricks and are still unable to sleep, maybe accept that you are not sleeping, soften your grasping for sleep, and embrace that you are just resting (which sometimes helps you fall asleep!).

Deb's story

I come from a long line of anxious women. There is no question that I carry a genetic predisposition for anxiety. I was very aware of my mother's irrational fears in early childhood and made a commitment to myself that I would not allow fear to contain me. I look at that fiercely spirited and rebellious girl, who is still a part of me, with deep respect and gratitude. I made wise choices with my friendships and romantic relationships in childhood and adolescence, so I was able to remain true to myself, which supported a healthy nervous system.

In college, my naive and trusting heart led to experiences that left me with lots of reasons to relate to the "me too" movement, including a sexual assault that I kept secret. Still, I had good instincts, and I healed my nervous system by spending time in nature and being with friends who kept me grounded and reminded me that I was loved and safe. Later on, I sought out therapy and somatic practices to address my trauma.

I did not get stuck in dysregulation until I became a single mom when my sons were 18 months and 5 years of age. I needed to quickly find full-time work and take care of my very young children on my own. I was overwhelmed and unable to function. I experienced pretty much all of the symptoms on the dysregulation list, including insomnia, digestive issues, anxiety, and a sense of hypervigilance. But, thanks to my circle of friends, family, and colleagues, I found my way through but my nervous system remained easily dysregulated.

I credit my fabulous therapist and somatic practitioners, the love of my children, dear friends, my mindfulness practices, and solace in the outdoors for my return to health and well-being and my ability to learn to regulate my nervous system. Over the years, I've benefited greatly from:

- Committing to a more consistent meditation, spiritual, and writing practices
- My developed a self-compassion practice
- Started Practicing yoga, ultimately training to be a yoga teacher
- Connection with friends and family, giving and receiving attention, love, and care
- White water kayaking

- Joy of music and dance in my daily life
- Acupuncture when I entered perimenopause
- A love of gardening and getting my hands in the earth
- Living with pets.

Each of these aspects of my life required me to prioritize my well-being and sometimes that felt impossible, especially when my children were still at home. I was able to create practices with varying levels of consistency in my life. Some have been more on and off than others. Now that I am postmenopausal and my children are adults, I realize that slowly, almost imperceptibly, I found my way back to what feels like my girlhood self.

My body, my spiritual life, my beloveds, and nature have been with me all along and helped me find my way. Meeting my body, listening to and respecting my body have been steadfast. Yes, my mother's declining health, politics, and other hard things that are simply part of a human life challenge and trigger me. But overall, I can honestly say I find regulating my nervous system and responding rather than reacting to life's tricky bits more accessible. I can more easily accept the messy and the hard parts while I look for the glimmers, set boundaries, and allow myself to dance, write, and to rest.

The intersection of nervous system regulation, sleep, and nourishment

In this chapter, you've learned how your body's nervous system becomes dysregulated, how you might regulate yourself, and the importance of rest and good sleep habits to support your nervous system and well-being. I want to focus more on how these factors affect how you nourish and care for your body in midlife and beyond.

Our world can feel overwhelming and unjust. Life itself can be unpredictable, and midlife and beyond is a time when we typically face increasing changes, transitions, and surprises, including those our bodies are experiencing. The longer we live, the more challenging our experiences are, and the older we are, the more likely we are to feel marginalized in our youth-obsessed culture. Difficulties and traumas cause all of us to experience varying degrees of dysregulated nervous systems, making rest and sleep more elusive.

Traumas of any degree, nervous system dysregulation, and disordered eating behaviors are commonly intertwined. Remember, disordered eating thoughts and behaviors are protective and, many times, attempts to cope with your life's traumas and stresses. One of the trickiest aspects of these patterns is that disordered eating behaviors tend to provide a sense of familiarity and, therefore, security and comfort at a time when precisely those feelings are so needed. In other words, eating disorder behaviors often serve as a way to achieve a sense of embodied safety and protection, which is what you may feel midlife is ultimately robbing you of! It is important to understand this catch-22. The very thing you may find comforting initially may also be the thing that harms you and makes you feel much worse in the long run.

Understanding your vulnerability to disordered eating behaviors and diet/wellness/anti-aging during this chapter of life, turning away from these seductive and ultimately harmful patterns while turning toward caring for your nervous system with permission to rest and sleep well, is what I hope you are interested in. This is a practice for your lifetime, so please know that it will not be fast or perfect. Turning toward daily practices to support your nervous system will change your life and protect you from lapsing into disordered eating, aka diet/wellness culture mess.

With these transformative steps of Part 1 and Part 2 behind you, Part 3 will invite you to thrive and see midlife and beyond as a time of emergence.

3
THRIVING

Midlife and beyond as emergence

9

Intimacy, body image, and embodiment in midlife and beyond

Have you seen the much-loved film *Good Luck to You, Leo Grande*? If you haven't, I highly recommend it! The 2022 film centers on the journey of a woman who is widowed and retired, played by Emma Thompson, who was 64 years old at the time of filming. To explore intimacy and reclaim her sense of self after a lifetime of unsatisfying sex and repression, she hires Leo Grande, a young, sensitive, and charming sex worker. The story unfolds over their encounters in a hotel room, showcasing their evolving relationship. At the same time, she becomes reacquainted with her body, awakening to the possibilities of pleasure and empowered to ask for what she desires. The exploration and unfolding wonder of her body seems like a third character in the film.

The powerful final scene of the film shows 64-year-old Emma Thompson gazing into the full-length mirror, her naked body reflecting back at her. Her expression shifts from a look of criticism to discomfort to timid curiosity and finally to a friendly, playful, and even confident smile.

I am re-making this film in my imagination, wondering how this story would go if the mirror-gazing experience occurred at the *beginning* rather than the end. What would it be like to prioritize your own gaze and befriend your body before you concern yourself with the gaze of another? Or have we been so conditioned to look at our bodies or objectify ourselves that we can only relate to our bodies as reflected in the gaze of another?

This chapter revisits the cultural influences on your relationship with and perception of your body in midlife and beyond, primarily related to intimacy and sexuality. You'll also explore how objectifying yourself disrupts intimate connection and how embodiment supports healthy connection and pleasure. You'll learn practices that support your embodied intimacy as a way to encourage your sexual satisfaction and empowerment based on your unique preferences in midlife and beyond.

In my nearly 40 years of navigating the terrain of body criticism and judgment with clients, the effect body image has on intimacy and sexuality is among the most common concerns discussed in sessions. Sometimes, these conversations are rooted in recent body-shaming comments from a loved one or a stranger. Sometimes, comments from decades ago stir up painful body criticism, shame, trauma, disconnection, and dissociation.

The good news is sometimes clients discuss their newfound excitement about intimacy due to increased body confidence and growth toward a greater capacity for embodiment, body acceptance, and greater trust in their bodies. Is there anything sexier than being comfortable in your body?

It may also be true that midlife events and experiences decrease your interest in intimacy, and that's okay, too. There is no right or wrong way to have a body or to experience intimacy and sexuality as long as there is consent. What genuinely matters is the intimacy you are interested in experiencing—or not. Sometimes, your partner's desires may also invite more curiosity and exploration of your body and what brings you pleasure.

As sex therapist Anna Fleig, LCMHC, CST, MDiv, MA, said when I interviewed her for this chapter, "Satisfying sex begins with your relationship with yourself and your own body. We are all responsible for our own desire."

Your sexual interest and comfort with intimacy are affected by multiple factors, including familial and cultural conditioning, your life, your body story, your well-being and energy, feeling safe, heard, and understood, self-awareness, sexual body awareness, and your capacity for embodiment. Let's begin by looking at the cultural narratives we receive about our bodies, desires, intimacy, and sexuality.

The body hierarchy and beauty

Let's revisit the body hierarchy from Chapter 4 and, more specifically, how this cultural stratification of bodies affects our perception of beauty, body image, and intimacy. Every culture has a beauty ideal, though the details vary. In the Western world, the ideal body is the young, white, thin, and able body with a long list of other traits, such as being hairless, curvy in all the right places, yet otherwise toned, defined, muscular or fit, to mention the most common attributes we've been conditioned to associate with a sexy body. The list continues with flawless skin, thick, typically straight, long hair, and on and on it goes. Remember, this cultural narrative is a fiction upheld by several different hundred-billion and trillion-dollar industries that profit from your self-criticism and belief that your perfectly amazing body is not enough.

If you're missing any of those traits associated with the beauty ideal, you may see your body as "flawed." To further complicate your perception of your body, the changes experienced in midlife and beyond likely mean the loss of attributes you once associated with feeling sexy or fuckable. You may believe you're expected to do everything within your power to conform to this beauty ideal, but this is what we call a "limiting belief," meaning if you believe your body is inadequate and no longer sexy, it limits your capacity to feel comfortable in your body sexually.

Your body, and its perceived fuckability, is not your value

Many women see menopause as a threshold opening to becoming "unfuckable." For some, that is honestly a relief. For some, this change is experienced as a tragic loss. Think Blanche in the show

The Golden Girls. I am grateful that our culture is beginning to talk more openly about the experiences of menopause. I'm hopeful this destigmatization will empower you to discover your interest in remaining sexy, or not, just as you are. Your body, your choice.

However you choose to navigate intimacy in midlife+, be curious about how you perceive your body: see the difference between what you experience as beautiful and sexy and what culture upholds and defines as beautiful and sexy. We've been sold a narrow version of beauty for so long, questioning it means wading through a mountain of bullshit just to figure out what you actually see as beautiful. Remember, you are exposed to hundreds of images every day that not only fit a narrow beauty ideal but are likely filtered, photoshopped, and may even be an image created by AI. We only see diverse bodies if we seek them out. Sources of images of diverse bodies are included in the Resources section.

Zoom out. When you peel back the layers of what you've been conditioned to see as beautiful and sexy, recognize that what you define as beautiful and sexy is unique to you. Beauty is an aspect of the natural world, and that includes you. Beauty is there for you to notice when you can slow down and recognize it as such. It's in the bark of trees exposed to decades of the elements that remind me of the skin on my hands; it's in the face of those you love when they belly laugh; it's in the slanty autumn golden light; it's in the swirl of lavender clouds in the early morning sky; it's the many colors exposed in the rocks cut away by hundreds of years by the power of the river. Sometimes, the sight of beauty takes our breath away or inspires an abrupt inhale of the awe of what's before you. What you perceive as beautiful is unique to you and brings an element of richness to your life. When we notice it, it enriches our lives.

Time is an artist

Your ability to see the beauty in your body as you age relies on the story you are carrying about your body and aging, which has been learned. You may have grown up with people recognizing and speaking about your beauty, along with your many other attributes. I sure hope you were affirmed for a multitude of your traits, in addition to your beauty.

You may have grown up believing beauty as essential to feeling loved; therefore, it is another complicated pressure in your life. You may have far too much heard body criticism, making your relationship with your body especially challenging; I am sorry if that happened to you. **You are your own unique, beautiful self, and the passing of time does not take that away.**

If you are having a hard time believing this right now, it is because the beauty, diet, and anti-aging industrial complexes have gotten under your skin and in your head. They've got you thinking about your body as not enough or too much, or just plain wrong. Feeling insecure in your body is understandable in a world that undermines you. And the insecurity you feel profits multiple industries! You've been lied to, maybe for your whole life, but *especially* from midlife and beyond.

However, I'll bet you can see beauty in others. Remember, this is not about making yourself mirror what you've been told fits the idea of what is beautiful. Is there any part of you that *knows* you are beautiful in that much more expansive, honest, and real kind of way you see in nature?

This means you don't have to do anything to fix yourself; you don't have to work on yourself and your body to fit the beauty ideal. Your mission, if you choose to accept it, is to be in partnership with your body and become more embodied in this next act of your life. Your mission is **not** to change how your body looks so you feel better about how your body looks. Rather it is to explore how you can thrive in your reclaimed partnership with your body—including intimacy. But what does that even look like?

You are invited to be in your body, or embodied, and spend time there, for in a moment of quiet, protected from the noise and pressure of the beauty/diet/anti-aging industrial complexes. Both thriving and intimacy are about turning toward our internal experience with presence, curiosity, and compassion.

One of my favorite teachers is John O'Donohue, the Irish poet and philosopher, whose words about beauty ring true for me:

> "Beauty isn't all about just nice loveliness. Beauty is about more rounded, substantial becoming. So I think beauty in that sense is about an emerging fullness, a greater sense of grace and elegance, a deeper sense of depth, and also a kind of homecoming for the enriched memory of your unfolding life."

So recognizing your own beauty—**true beauty**, not the **idea** of glamour or beauty—is nothing more or less than awakening to your unfolding and homecoming. In this quiet shift, you realize you belong just as you are. In moments like these, you will be able to see your beauty and be open to intimacy with your experience despite the stories you've been told. Fuck the patriarchy! I was delighted to be able to interview Karen Walrond about her thoughts:

Notes from an expert

Karen Walrond, Afro-Trinidadian author of *Radiant Rebellion: Reclaim Aging, Practice Joy, and Raise a Little Hell*:

> The woman that you see across the room that you're like, wow! She's beautiful.
>
> What attracts us often has little to do with whether or not she looks like a runway model. What we tend to react to might be some of her physicality. But it's also her movement. That's not her static standing there. It's the way she moves. It's the way she laughs. It's the way she expresses herself. We don't react to each other based on a static image. We're drawn to each other because of the energy we have and how we move through the world. That's what really turns us on about each other.

> My idea of beauty is so much more about how I want to show up in a room. What do I want people to feel when they're around me, and what do I want people to think of themselves when they're around me? That's far more interesting to me.
>
> When I was in my twenties, when I walked into a room, I wanted a man to see me and immediately be attracted to me based on my appearance. Now, I would love to walk into a room and for people to still be attracted to me. And then, when I leave, for them to not understand why and wonder if there was something about my brain, what I said, and the way that I felt great about myself because of the conversation we had. She was generous and warm. I want them to think, 'What was that? Why am I so attracted to this person?' Yeah, I love that. I want to do that until I'm a hundred years old.

Andrea's story

Andrea reached out to schedule her first session with me after hearing another of my clients describe her experience.

Andrea was 45 years old and had been on diets ever since the third grade, when her mother took her to Weight Watchers. Andrea had tried several very aggressive, restrictive liquid diets administered at a medical center and multi-disciplinary behavioral plans, which required her to journal extensively about every morsel she ate. Andrea had honestly tried everything except gastric bypass surgery, which she refused. She was successful in her career and all other aspects of her life. Andrea described her weight as the only thing she had not been successful with.

As I got to know Andrea, I discovered her thoughts and behaviors had been mired in anorexic patterns for many years. Unbeknownst to Andrea, she had been struggling with ARFID (Avoidant/Restrictive Food Intake Disorder) since she was a child. Even though she found many foods repulsive, her parents insisted that she eat what the family ate. To make matters worse, her mother was a chronic dieter and only made bland, unappetizing meals. So, Andrea learned to dissociate when eating to "just get through it."

Her therapist and I diagnosed her with "atypical anorexia," which she found to be hard to believe but also made perfect sense to her.

With this development, Andrea was highly motivated to learn more about relating to her body with less fat phobia and more body respect. She fell in love with this aspect of our work together and became a student of all things body liberation.

As she continued to do the work, her depression lifted, and she became much more comfortable in her body. She described much-improved intimacy with her partner, saying she felt they were more in love than ever. They decided to vacation during their next anniversary and renew their vows. Listening to Andrea describe her unfolding toward more body neutrality, then acceptance, then respect, and even caring for her body as her capacity for embodiment, intimacy, and sexuality blossomed made me wonder which was coming first sometimes. Was her ability to feel embodied and experience intimacy and pleasure supporting her eating disorder recovery or vice versa? Or maybe it was all parts of her mending her relationship with her body from different angles. It was a gift to witness the process of her liberation.

Of course, there were challenges along the way; there were periods of fatigue during the process. Working toward embodiment, reconnecting with her body's sensations, and learning to trust her body again required commitment to prioritizing her internal experience rather than following external rules, which took time. Over the years, Andrea has blossomed, inhabiting her body respectfully and much more confidently. As of this writing, she reports that her sexual intimacy is tracking with her body connection, or embodiment, and confidence and is also much improved. We continue to work on complex eating issue sand she is also committed to moving her body more and is now working with a fat-positive personal trainer.

Now that you are well on your way to unlearning stories that limit your body's connection and confidence, let's turn our attention to your embodiment.

Embodiment

Connecting to your body contributes to your well-being and resilience. If you are attuned to your bodily experiences, this opens up your capacity to be present and awake to your own experience and connect to others.

One of my preferred sources for learning about embodiment is Hillary McBride, Ph.D., author of *Embodiment and Eating Disorders: Theory, Research, Prevention, and Treatment*. Dr. McBride defines embodiment as "the experience of the body as engaged in the world, being fully present with the experience of being in our body."

However, many potential barriers exist to your ability to be embodied, including:

- The messages you've received about your body, which result in you looking at your body as an object to be judged
- Your experiences, especially trauma
- Previous dieting or disordered eating, which require you to disconnect from your body and ignore your hunger
- Your neurological differences such as anxiety, ADHD, or autism, which may or may not contribute to experiencing your body differently
- Avoiding uncomfortable emotions.

Objectifying and judging your body make it very difficult to be embodied. If you judge your body, you may struggle to be present and connected to your body while having sexual experiences with yourself or others. This disconnection can complicate or disrupt your enjoyment and interest in sexual intimacy.

But for a moment let's revisit the first factor: *the messages you've received about your body*. Grind culture and modern lifestyle in Western society make it difficult, if not impossible, to feel embodied. Our culture celebrates and applauds the mind's dominance over our bodies, encouraging us to ignore our body's requests for rest, pleasure, and nourishment.

Many clients tell me that nourishing themselves in the middle of the day is one of their most significant challenges because "nobody around here takes lunch." We run errands, catch up on emails, or simply work through our lunch hours. Can you relate? You may not take the time to drink beverages throughout the day, either. My clients, who are teachers and healthcare workers, often tell me they hesitate to stay hydrated at work because they cannot take a break to go to the restroom. As you might imagine, this contributes to dehydration, urinary tract infections, and kidney and bladder damage over time. There is a cost to how our institutions require us to ignore our bodies and their wisdom.

These sorts of experiences and beliefs disconnect you from your body. If they become a habit, you lose the ability to notice or access your body's sensations, desires, and needs. This creates barriers to your embodiment and, therefore, aspects of your sexual experiences.

In my nearly 40 years of hearing body stories, I've been curious about how my clients experience embodiment and body relationships. Some describe their body relationship as adversarial; maybe they struggle with chronic pain and feel like their body has betrayed them. As we heard from Andrea, maybe being with their body is confusing and anxiety-provoking so a part of them learned to protect them by disconnecting or dissociating. Past traumas can make the body feel like it's not a safe place to be. Slowly, with complete reminders that it is your choice and entirely up to when you are ready, discovering ways to become safely connected to your body, or embodied, again is a crucial component of mending your relationship with your body.

The best starting point is to allow yourself to approach your relationship with your body with kindness, compassion, curiosity, respect, and as much playfulness as possible. According to sex therapist Dr. Cheyenne Carter, LCMHC, CST, solo sexual experiences sexual aids and erotica can help you explore and get to know your body, sexuality, and preferences. She concludes: "Sexual aids and erotica are helpful and empowering and need to be demystified and destigmatized in our culture." Here are some practices that help you approach your relationship with your body with kindness. As always, take what helps and leave the rest. You may want to mark this page as something you would like to return to when you are ready.

Practices

Mirror gazing (part 1)

Set aside a time to look at yourself in as close to a full-size mirror as you are comfortable with in as little clothing as you are comfortable with. As you gaze at yourself, take note of the parts of your body that you are fond of. Tell yourself what you like about those parts. If there are parts that you are not fond of, see if you can find neutral acceptance of those parts. Use this as a practice that you engage in with the intention to move toward more and more acceptance, kindness, and care. When you notice a more critical thought, zoom out and become curious about where you learned that and maybe even say to yourself, "Who says?!" The more you practice this ritual with the intention to hold your body in a rosy glow, the more you will soften your criticism and find body neutrality and care for your body, one day!

Mirror gazing (part 2)

Psychologists have been researching the effects of this practice, in which subjects gaze at their reflection for 10 to 15 minutes in a meditative state cultivating a kind intention toward themselves, allowing them to see how their thoughts affect them through changes in their facial expressions.

In other words, in being present with their feelings, they're exposed to a de-objectified perspective of their image, seeing themselves as they might see a beloved person in their lives. Researchers found that in eight sessions over ten days, the meditators reported decreased stress, depression, and anxiety and a significant increase in self-compassion levels. Subjects who did this meditation regularly generally reported feeling more comfortable with their appearance.

What if when you look in the mirror, you see not an object to judge but a wise and caring human, the way you see the people you love?

Awareness of your self-talk

Developing awareness of the way you are talking to yourself is an essential practice. If you feel like you are not aware of your inner dialogue, you may want to check in with yourself and notice what you were just thinking and feeling several times a day.

My favorite recommendation is to pair a new habit with something in your life that is firmly in place, such as checking in with yourself when you wake up, again for at least three meals or snacks, and again before going to sleep. Ask yourself, "What was I thinking, feeling, or saying to myself just now?" This practice requires you to slow down and stay more connected to yourself as you go through your day. This is more challenging than it sounds, so there is no reason to expect perfection here! Whatever starts to unfold for you is enough. Change happens in small steps over time.

As a side note, if you've been disconnected from your body through being rushed, multitasking, distracted, or dissociated (which we all do to some degree), the process of connecting may be uncomfortable for you. Please trust yourself and remember that you're doing the best you can. Remember, resistance is usually protective so please be gentle with yourself.

Importance of self-compassion

If I had to pick one non-negotiable practice, it would be self-compassion. This one is a must! Starting to do the practices above brings up thoughts and feelings of body judgment and shame, so it is essential that you have the skills to care for yourself with self-compassion.

Shame causes you to drop anchor and get stuck in cycles of "all or nothing." Self-compassion gives you the energy to keep moving forward and the space to become curious about your experience. You may find Dr. Kristen Neff's work helpful if you need some ideas. See the Resources section for more. Sometimes these practices can start to feel too heavy and serious. Carrying all of this lightly keeps this process sustainable. So, let's switch gears and get playful.

Embodied play

Do you have memories of playing when you were a kid? This may be a rich jumping-off point for creating more play in your life. If you don't remember, try looking at old photographs or interviewing your friends and family about what they remember. Play that connects you with your body may include throwing a frisbee, skipping, hula hooping, swinging on a swing, dancing, riding a bike or scooter, playing a game like Twister, finger painting, or water play. It could also be playful to simply go outdoors and play in the sprinkler or walk in the rain. Play allows you to connect with your body in a way that helps lighten the process.

Healing your relationship with your body is challenging and effortful. Sprinkling in some play may provide comic relief and allow you to carry this lightly.

Wake up to your senses

Turn your attention to each of your senses. Close your eyes or rest your gaze and notice the feeling of air or a breeze or the sun on your skin. Notice the feeling of your clothing on your skin or the temperature of your glass or cup in your hands.

Use essential oils, aromatic soaps, or scented candles to engage your sense of smell.

When you are eating, slow down and savor your food. Pretend you need to describe this experience to a Martian or write a poem about your experience. What words come to mind?

Take a few minutes to notice all you can hear around you, then farther away, stretching your hearing out in all directions.

What colors can you see from where you are at this moment? Are any particular textures noticeable? What catches your eye's attention? Engaging your senses is an accessible bridge into being embodied. Remember to let your life gently remind you to practice, practice, practice.

Relationships take time

Getting to know your body is like cultivating a healthy relationship with the ultimate goal of befriending your body. Rushing relationships just doesn't work. Experiment with the practices I've mentioned here or some of your own to feel more connected and at ease in your body.

As you build this relationship, you will also develop a greater degree of respect for your own body. Worrying about the judgment of others will likely begin to fade. And as my wise client said: "And obviously, the right people aren't going to care."

"Take your time" sounds just like "I love you" to me. *Please take your time.*

Body respect and acceptance and more capacity for embodiment may open up and perhaps deepen your sexual intimacy, starting with yourself. As my friend Anna Fleig, a sex therapist, says, "I am always a great date with myself."

Embodied intimacy

Embodiment plays a significant role in how you experience sexual intimacy, especially in midlife and beyond when your body's sexual response is changing, requiring more time and plenty of lube! When you're embodied—fully connected to and aware of your body—you're more attuned to sensations, desires, and comfort levels, which can deepen your sexual intimacy. Here are some ways embodiment influences your sexual experiences:

- *Sensory awareness*: Being embodied allows you to be more aware of sensations and cues, heightening your pleasure and responsiveness. This awareness can make your experiences more vivid and pleasurable as you increase your capacity to be present and connected to your body and your partner's.

- *Body acceptance*: Embodiment encourages you to accept your body as it is, pushing back against the disconnect that comes with thinking your body should fit societal ideals and standards. This acceptance can soften your inhibitions, allowing you to connect with yourself and your partner with less fear of judgment or body shame.

- *Asking for what you want*: When you are present and connected to your body, you are more capable of identifying what you want and then voicing your wants, needs, and desires. This presence, clarity, and empowerment may foster more satisfying sexual intimacy, as both you and your partner can more openly express your wishes and boundaries with greater openness.

- *Drop the pressure*: Embodiment helps shift the focus away from appearance or "performance" toward personal experience and sensation. This mindset supports a relaxed, less goal-oriented approach to intimacy, which can increase satisfaction.

- *Heightened emotions and intimacy*: Being present with your body and bodily sensations will likely increase your awareness of your emotions. With this increased sensitivity, you may experience a deeper connection and vulnerability with your body, yourself, and your partner. This openness may allow for greater intimacy and trust, strengthening the emotional aspect of your sexual experiences.

- *Rolling with change*: As your body and your partner's body shift and change with the passage of time, increasing awareness and access to connection with your body can help you adapt. As you age, one of the truths about your brain is that you have an increased capacity for adapting to change. You can adjust to new rhythms, body changes, and needs with more connection to your body. Embodiment allows you to explore what brings you pleasure in new and different ways.

The practices we've covered, such as mindfulness, body-focused therapies, and movement practices, promote embodiment and may potentially enhance your sexual wellness, body confidence, and intimacy.

With the potential support of embodied intimacy in your life, how do the changes in midlife and beyond affect your sexual experiences?

Sexuality in midlife and beyond

Emily Nagoski, PhD, highly respected sex educator and author of the much-loved books *Come as You Are: The Surprising New Science That Will Transform Your Sex Life*, describes the common midlife narrative as a time "when apparently, every hormone we ever had floats away on a sea of aging and we are left sexless and neutered to hold hands at sunset."

But despite the commonly held ageist, ableist, and fat-phobic narrative that sexuality is a privilege designed only for the young, thin, fit, and physically healthy, research continues to reveal a very different story—that the majority of us maintain an interest in sexual intimacy and can engage in satisfying sexual experiences of all kinds until the end of our lives.

Just like there is no right or wrong way to have a body, there is no right or wrong way to be a sexual being.

Yes, midlife and beyond brings myriad barriers and challenges to satisfying sexual experiences:

- Hormonal shifts, such as those that occur during menopause or andropause, can lead to changes like vaginal dryness, reduced libido, or erectile challenges. Joint pain, muscle stiffness, or fatigue can also change your sexual experiences.
- Anxiety and stress may intensify during midlife as you face transitions like career changes, empty nesting, parenting adult children, or caring for aging parents, which can affect your enthusiasm for intimacy.

- Long-term relationships can experience sexual ruts, communication challenges, or unresolved conflicts over the years, which may alter intimacy and satisfaction.
- The myth that sex is less relevant or desirable in midlife+ often contributes to dismissing or ignoring your desires. Inadequate information on sexual health for midlife and beyond can also be a barrier to exploring sexual intimacy, although this seems to be improving!
- Your needs and what brings you pleasure have likely evolved, sometimes leading to misalignment with your partner's needs and pleasures if they're not openly communicated.
- Chronic illness and other medical issues may affect your interest in, and your body's response to, intimacy. The good news is that we are highly capable of adaptation as we age. This is another opportunity to be curious about yourself and expand your definition of intimacy.
- How you feel about your body in midlife and beyond need not be on this list!

Explore these barriers with patience and open-mindedness to overcome challenges, rediscover pleasure, and cultivate fulfilling, exciting sexual intimacy. Or not! Again, there is no pressure here. If you are interested, here are some ideas about meeting your challenges:

- Many find relief and improved comfort by using lubricants, considering hormone replacement options, especially vaginal estrogen creams, or engaging in regular movement, especially activities that support a healthy pelvic floor, to maintain the physical stamina and flexibility that may support your sexual intimacy. See more about pelvic floor health in Chapter 7 and the Resources section.
- Managing health conditions with the guidance of healthcare providers, discussing medication side effects, and exploring

alternative treatments where possible can help minimize the impact on your sexual well-being.

- Practices like mindfulness, therapy, or stress management skills can improve your emotional health and reduce the possibility that stress and overwhelm may be affecting your capacity for sexual intimacy.

- Talk about it! Having brave and vulnerable conversations with partners can relieve relational stress and significantly improve intimacy. Open communication, couples counseling, educating yourself, and a willingness to mix it up and explore new ways of connecting (from date nights to trying new things in the bedroom) can help reinvigorate your sexual intimacy with yourself and your partner and potentially increase your pleasure and satisfaction. Embracing open discussions with partners about evolving preferences can help you and your partner adapt, feel supported, and stay connected. This process can make your intimacy more pleasurable by acknowledging changes rather than resisting them.

- Reading age-positive, body liberation, and sex-positive resources, joining communities focused on empowered aging and body diversity, and seeking inclusive healthcare providers can offer new perspectives and tools for sexual well-being. Yay to you for picking up this book! There are more in the Resources section, too.

- Focusing on self-acceptance, embracing age-affirming and body-respecting narratives, and prioritizing embodiment practices can help you positively reconnect with your and your partner's changing bodies, making intimacy feel safer and more accessible.

By the way, it bears mentioning that many remain unaware of the increased risk factors for sexually transmitted infections (STIs), including HIV infection via lack of knowledge, changes in the vaginal lining, and declines in immune function. Estimates suggest that by the year 2030, more than half of all individuals living with HIV will be over the age of 50. As a recent billboard that made its rounds on social media clearly stated: STIs are not ageist!

Dating in midlife+

Full transparency: At the time of this writing, I am 66 years old and single, and I am taking a break from dating, primarily to write this book. This was the reason for ending my last relationship because it became clear that we were in different places. He was ready to retire, and I was not interested in retirement at all.

Being single in midlife+ is a specific type of challenge related to body image, so I want to make sure we address it. One of my most popular posts on my Instagram account addressed body image as a single woman dating over 60, so I know I am not alone! According to a 2022 Pew survey, around 30 percent of adults in the US over 50 are single. Of course, not all singles are interested in dating or being in a committed relationship. I count myself as one of the "Single over 60" who relishes independence even though I know there is a stigma about being single at my age. This is also starting to change, and I'm adding my voice to that conversation!

In a 2022 study published in *Psychology of Aging*, singles in midlife and older were less likely than their younger counterparts to say they wanted to date or find a romantic relationship, and people's satisfaction with being single tends to jump in middle age. Dr. Bella DePaulo, author of *Single at Heart: The Power, Freedom, and Heart-filling Joy of the Single Life*, says, "People in their 60s and beyond who are single and flourishing is an untold story. And it's a feel-good story that shatters all of our stereotypes."

According to a study published in 2018 in the *Journal of the American Psychological Association*, self-esteem peaks at age 60 and holds steady at this lifetime peak through age 70. I'm hoping with the help of the anti-ageism movement, this would hold far beyond 70 too. Don't forget, aging is not the problem, ageism is!

Dating in midlife and beyond can be a rewarding but complex experience. At this stage in your life, after spending time focused on your career, family, and other pursuits, you may find that your social circle is smaller than when you were younger. You can join new activities like taking classes, attending workshops, or volunteering to meet people in a low-pressure environment. Reach out to old friends or colleagues. They may introduce you to others.

The years that brought you to this stage in life have helped you clarify what you want in a relationship, which is a strength. However, it can also cause you to be more selective, which narrows the pool of potential dates. It's wise to be selective!

If you are in midlife+, you are probably juggling your career, caregiving for family or friends, or even parenting teens or adult children. Finding the time and energy for dating may require some soul-searching and discernment. The best bet is to communicate your concerns about time and energy honestly and early. Be upfront about your commitments and what time you can realistically dedicate to a relationship.

If you haven't dated in years, the lay of the land may have changed quite a bit. Navigating online dating apps and modern dating etiquette can feel like a lot. Muster your confidence and approach online dating keeping in mind that this is optional and there is no rush. Apps like Silver Singles, Date My Age or OurTime cater to midlife+ daters. AARP (formerly the American Association of Retired Persons) keeps its review post about these apps up to date so that is worth an internet search. Make your profile authentic and up to date, highlighting your passions, humor, and what makes you unique. Stay cautious while optimistic. Be mindful of red flags, like anyone who is pushy and rushing the process or asking for personal information. When your connection passes your tests, approach your new potential date with an open heart.

Since we become more unique as we age, we have a range of relationship expectations and lifestyle preferences in midlife and beyond. Some seek serious, long-term, committed relationships, while others prioritize companionship or casual connections. Compatibility can be more challenging at this stage in life. Carefully define your priorities and be clear about what you want. Whether it's a serious relationship or casual dating, knowing your goals helps you communicate effectively and set boundaries.

Try to be open-minded. While it's good to know your deal-breakers, flexibility can open doors to surprising connections. This chapter of your life may be a good time to broaden your horizons.

Take small steps as you open yourself to vulnerability. Start with low-stakes interactions like casual coffee dates or a walk in a public park. Remind yourself that vulnerability is key to building trust and potentially intimate connections of all kinds.

As we discussed earlier, societal beauty standards and internalized ageism may contribute to feeling insecure about dating again. Continue to challenge social narratives about "good bodies" and cultivate age-affirming social media accounts representing diverse bodies to help you to reframe how you see yourself. Embrace your unique beauty just as you are.

Despite these challenges, dating in this season of life can also be incredibly fulfilling if you choose to jump in. At this stage in life, you are more self-aware, emotionally mature, and better equipped to engage in healthy relationships. Now, you have a better understanding of what you are looking for, what you will and will not tolerate, and you are more confident in expressing what you know about yourself to your potential partners.

Again, dating in midlife and beyond is **optional**. There is no right or wrong way to age, have a body, date, or have sex. There is only discovering the way aging in your body, just as you are deciding to date or experience sexual intimacy your way. You have value regardless of your body's size, age, ability, gender, or sexual preference.

Whatever you choose to do about dating and sexual intimacy is absolutely up to you. The goal is to enjoy your life and cultivate satisfaction and pleasure in whatever way you decide. If you choose to date, reclaim your narrative and let go of the narratives you may hear from those around you. Dating at any age is a testament to your openness and vitality—be proud of it!

- *Enjoy the process*: Not every date will lead to a relationship, but each experience can teach you something.

- *Celebrate your independence*: Midlife dating is about finding someone who enhances your life, not completes it.

Take some time to discern what you are looking for when it comes to dating, sexual intimacy, and your values and intentions.

Journal prompts for dating in midlife+

These questions are for you if you are single and considering dating. Here are a few questions to get you started. Taking the time to reflect on these questions can help you approach dating with intention, clarity, and more confidence.

Am I ready to date?

- Am I emotionally ready? Have I healed from past relationships or experiences that might affect my ability to be open and present in a new one?
- Do I feel confident and comfortable in my own company? Do I want to learn to enjoy my company before seeking a relationship? Am I seeking a relationship out of loneliness, or am I happy with myself and ready to share my life with someone else?

- What does a fulfilling relationship look like for me? Do I know the type of connection, values, and companionship I desire?

- Do I have the time and energy to invest in dating? Do I have time for myself and care for myself the way I would like, and do I have enough time and energy to add dating to the mix? Can I balance dating with other commitments, relationships, and enjoyment in my life?

- Exactly what am I looking for in a relationship? Am I seeking companionship, romance, a life partner, or something else?

- Am I clear on my dealbreakers and non-negotiables? What values, habits, or characteristics are essential or unacceptable to me in a partner, and can I handle setting boundaries and communicating these issues if I need to?

- Am I open to new experiences? How willing am I to try new things and explore dating outside of my usual type or approach? Or am I clear that I am looking for familiar situations and experiences?

- Am I prepared for the emotional ups and downs of dating? Do I have the capacity to navigate rejection, disappointment, or uncertainty if they arise?

- How do I want to show up in a relationship? What qualities or behaviors do I want to bring to a potential partnership, and am I ready to share these parts of myself?

- How does dating align with my personal goals? Does finding a partner or companion align with my goals for independence, career, travel, or other personal pursuits?

- What does "success" look like in dating for me? Is it finding "the one," enjoying the experience of meeting new people, or something else?

- How will I know I'm ready to start? What specific feelings, circumstances, or mindset will signal to me that it's the right time to start dating?

I hope taking the time to reflect on these questions helps you know more about your values, expectations, and boundaries so you can enjoy yourself!

Am I ready for intimacy?

Sexual intimacy is a deeply personal decision, and reflecting on your readiness can help you navigate it with more confidence and clarity. Here are some thoughtful questions to explore your feelings and preparedness for sexual intimacy in midlife and beyond. Try turning up your compassion and curiosity with yourself as you ponder these questions:

- Am I comfortable with my own body? Do I feel confident and accepting of my body as it is, or do I need more self-compassion and care in certain areas? Remember, there is no perfection here, and if you start to think that you need to make your body "right," please take a breath and remember this is about your relationship with your body, not making your body fit the "beauty ideal." If it sends you into a shame spiral, please return to Chapter 4.
- How do I feel about physical touch and closeness? Am I open to receiving and giving physical affection, or do I feel hesitant or unsure about this aspect of intimacy?
- Exactly why am I seeking sexual intimacy? Am I pursuing it out of genuine desire, connection, and curiosity, or am I feeling pressure from societal expectations, a partner, or my own insecurities? Please take your time and center your satisfaction. Dating and sexual intimacy are optional. You can opt out until you feel clear and interested. No pressure! You get to age the way you want to age, with or without sexual intimacy.
- Am I emotionally ready to be vulnerable? Sexual intimacy often involves a level of emotional exposure. Am I prepared to open up in this way?

- Do I feel safe and respected by the person I'm considering intimacy with? Do I trust my partner and feel comfortable, safe, valued, and accepted as I am?
- Am I comfortable communicating my needs, boundaries, and desires? Can I talk about sex and openly discuss consent, preferences, and expectations with my partner? Am I comfortable setting boundaries? Am I comfortable with centering my own pleasure and asking for what I want? Do I know what I want?
- Am I comfortable discussing how my body has changed? How do hormonal shifts, medical conditions, or other factors impact me and my comfort or preferences in sexual intimacy, and can I share this with a potential partner?
- What role does emotional connection play in my desire for intimacy? Do I need a strong emotional connection to feel comfortable with sexual intimacy, or am I open to more casual experiences?
- Amongst all of my feelings about sexuality, am I excited about the idea of exploring my sexuality? Does the thought of intimacy bring me joy, curiosity, and a sense of empowerment?

Taking the time to reflect on these questions can help you step into sexual intimacy feeling self-assured, empowered, and in tune with your desires and needs.

Overall journal prompts and body check-in

Here are some journal prompts to help you explore and deepen your relationship with your body and sexuality in this season of your life. These prompts encourage you to inquire with compassionate curiosity about your beliefs, attitudes, and desires that shape your relationship with your body and sexuality.

As always, I encourage you to check in to see if you are comfortable with these questions. Give yourself lots of permission to skip any questions that bring up judgment and criticism or trigger you in any way. Take what feels helpful and leave the rest.

By now, I hope you are well-practiced in checking in with your body and even beginning to feel comfortable doing so. Take the time to start with a body check-in and then reference what you feel in your body as you answer these questions. It may be helpful to refer back to your body story, too.

You can trust your body. Your body is a source of wisdom.

Body relationship

- What are three things I appreciate about my body at this stage in my life?
- How has my relationship with my body changed over the years? What were some key moments?
- What messages about aging and body image have I internalized, and how do they impact how I feel about my body now?
- How would I like to feel about my body? What small, kind practices invite this shift in how I feel in my body? Can I make time for these practices?
- How do I respond to seeing images of bodies that look like mine in media, art, or life? What does this tell me about my beliefs on beauty and worth? Can I expand my definition of beauty and worth? What would it look like for this definition to include my body?
- What aspects of my body do I tend to focus on? Are there areas I avoid? What's behind those tendencies? Are there opportunities to make changes in these tendencies so that I might feel less negative, more neutral or more caring about my body just as I am?
- How does feeling connected or disconnected from my body affect my relationships with others?
- What would I say to a friend being judgmental and critical about their body? How can I apply that compassion to myself?

Sexuality

- What messages about sexuality did I hear growing up, and how do they shape my views today?
- How have my sexual interests and desires evolved over time? What new possibilities or experiences would I like to explore?
- What does sexual pleasure and satisfaction mean to me in this season of life, and is it different from other times in my life?
- How comfortable am I talking about sexuality and intimacy with others, including my partner(s) or friends? Would having more open conversations be helpful to me?
- What do I appreciate about my sexuality or sensuality? What about sexual intimacy feels challenging, and why?
- How do I feel about the changes in my body and the way these changes affect sexual intimacy? What thoughts or practices may support feeling more comfortable with these changes?
- What brings me pleasure or makes me feel alive? Can I make more room for those experiences in my life? What would that look like?
- How do I connect with my body during intimate moments? How might I deepen that connection?

Body image and sexual intimacy

- How does my body image affect my sexual experiences? How does one impact the other?
- What would it look like to feel confident in my body and sexuality, just as I am? How might I cultivate these qualities and experiences?
- What would it feel like to completely accept my body as it is in intimate situations?
- What values do I want to carry into this season of my life regarding body image, pleasure, and sexual intimacy? How can I start living by those values now?

These prompts can be revisited to see how your perspectives evolve, offering a compassionate path toward your curious connection with your body relationship and sexual intimacy. Onward to body respect, exploration, and pleasure!

Steps toward mending your body relationship for sexual well-being

Does your relationship with your body interfere with your sexual well-being?

Is there a voice in your head telling you you need to work on your body before you start dating again?

Is there a moment of body shame when you notice someone looking at you? Or when you look at yourself?

Does a rush of body shame run through you when you're in bed with your partner, putting the brakes on thoughts of your pleasure?

If this is you, your body story may interrupt your capacity for embodied intimacy and damage your sexual well-being. But you can do something about it!

Throughout this book, I've encouraged you to take an inside-out approach toward caring for yourself, and that is just as true when you consider your sexual intimacy. Here is a summary that you may want to refer to. Choose one or two of these practices for your (mostly) daily life.

Please remember, when it comes to shifting your relationship with your body, it takes time, patience, and practice, practice, practice. These changes happen in small, incremental steps until you can finally step out of the shadow of what's been keeping you stuck in your body story.

Shift your focus to pleasure and sensation

When engaging in intimate moments, focus on what feels good rather than how you think you look. Bringing attention to sensations can help you feel more embodied and present, which often enhances your experience.

Practices like mindfulness and breathwork can help you tune into your body and enjoy touch, closeness, and connection without being distracted by self-critical thoughts.

Practice self-compassion and positive self-talk

Negative self-talk about your body often affects confidence in intimate settings. Try to counter these thoughts by practicing self-compassion and speaking to yourself as you would a friend. Affirmations that honor your body can also help, such as, "My body is worthy of pleasure," or "I am deserving of love and intimacy."

Embrace the imperfections and changes that come with age as part of your unique beauty, shifting your mindset from criticism to appreciation.

Engage in movement you enjoy

Moving your body in ways that feel good—not for appearance's sake but for pleasure, strength, and well-being—can improve body appreciation and boost confidence. Activities like dancing, yoga, or walking encourage you to feel connected with your body and celebrate its abilities.

Movement can also release endorphins, boost mood, and reduce stress, all of which contribute to a more positive self-image.

Create body-positive rituals

Rituals that make you feel comfortable and beautiful in your skin—such as taking a warm bath, moisturizing, our skin, applied with care and kindness, or wearing clothes that feel good—can cultivate a positive relationship with your body. These rituals reinforce the idea that your body is worthy of care and respect.

Incorporating sensual or sensory aspects, like scented candles or soft fabrics, can make these routines enjoyable and deepen your connection to your physical self.

Challenge cultural narratives and internalized beliefs

Reflect on how societal pressures and messages around aging, appearance, and body ideals impact your self-image. Recognizing these influences can help you separate external expectations from your own values.

Surround yourself with age-affirming, sex-positive media that celebrates diverse bodies, especially those that embrace the beauty of aging. Granted, this is not easy to find. I recommend collecting these images or passages when you encounter them as these are gems worth keeping!

Open communication with your partner(s)

Sharing your feelings with your partner(s) about body image and intimacy can be incredibly liberating. When partners understand your insecurities or needs, it often leads to increased sensitivity, empathy and intimacy. Practicing vulnerability with trusted partners can help you feel safer and more accepted, which may reduce body-image anxiety in intimate moments.

Explore sensuality beyond sexuality

Sexual well-being isn't just about sex; it's also about feeling connected to your body and sensual self. Activities like touching different textures, exploring new scents, or enjoying music can awaken your senses and remind you that your body is a source of pleasure and joy.

Cultivating this connection to your senses outside of the bedroom can build confidence and self-acceptance that positively impact intimacy.

Practice gratitude for your body

Taking time to appreciate what your body allows you to experience can shift your focus from judging your appearance to acknowledging gratitude. A simple gratitude practice could include writing down or reflecting on a few things your body supports, like hugging a loved one or savoring a sensory experience. Over time, this gratitude can foster a more expansive and compassionate view of your body and its value.

Seek support when needed

If your body image issues feel stuck or overwhelming, working with a therapist, especially one trained in body image, somatic or sex-positive approaches, can be incredibly helpful. They can provide guidance on how to reframe your self-critical thoughts and heal your relationship with your body.

Embrace embodiment practices

Practices like yoga, tai chi, or belly-dancing can help you connect more deeply with your body, inviting appreciation for your strength, resilience, and sensuality. Being fully "in" your body can lessen thoughts of self-consciousness and make you feel more confident and open in intimate situations.

Each of these strategies can help to heal your relationship with your body, boosting your curiosity and confidence so that you enhance your sense of sexual well-being at any age. Remember, bodies change and that's okay. Curiosity is often your best way to approach your changing body. You may need more but it's such a wise starting place. And as always, you are the expert of you, so forget about any rules about your body and intimacy. You know what works best for you!

10

Body liberation as your legacy

"I still remember my mother's Saturday morning weigh-ins, the click of the bathroom scale, followed by the tsk of her tongue and a deep sigh, communicating her disappointment in her body."

"The family story about my grandmother was that she 'ate like a bird,' and so did my mother. I started realizing the same was expected of me when I asked for seconds, and my mother said, just loud enough for me to hear, 'You need to keep it under control,' followed by a loud sigh."

"My mother was tall, thin, beautiful, and a fashion model before I was born. She put me on a diet when I was in the 3rd grade because my belly was a bit round. I soon started sneaking food and got caught in chronic dieting mixed with restrict – binge cycles until now, at the age of 56."

"My father criticized my mother's body when we were at home, and when we were out, he commented on other women's bodies, many times comparing their bodies to my mother's. Then when I was about 12 years old, he started poking me in the belly and giving me the side-eye. I've been fighting diet culture and body-shaming comments in my head ever since."

"My grandmother was a fabulous cook and baker. My clearest memories are of finally breaking my mother's strict food rules and keeping the treats I enjoyed with my grandmother our little secret. To this day, I crave the foods that I associate with visiting my grandmother when I am feeling blue, lonely, or overwhelmed—or any discomfort really. It's no surprise that eating these foods is all I can think about when I start a diet or wellness program."

Do any of these stories resonate with you? In my nearly 40 years of practice, the most common denominator is that my clients experienced their first body shaming and/or food rules at home from well-intended family members. No shame or blame; as you've learned, we've all internalized the dominant messages of diet culture and ageism. In this chapter, you'll return to the discussion that started in Chapter 1: how your family influenced your relationship with food and your body. You'll develop a deeper understanding of how intergenerational diet culture and the potential for trauma may show up in your life. You'll also learn how you can heal from the diet culture and body shame you've inherited by re-parenting yourself, including using skills from the powerful modality of Internal Family Systems (IFS). As always, I'm introducing options here. Please take what works and leave the rest.

Finally, the most challenging and worthwhile process is learning to heal the damage you may have passed down to those you love. Body liberation can be your legacy, and you can expand the definition of what it is like to have a "good" body for the next generations. If not now, when, right? So here we go.

Unpacking the mess: Body shame, ageism, and diet culture

The first section of this book invited you to inventory the body shame, ageism, and diet culture mess you had passed down to you, along with how these beliefs manifested in your body story. If you have been keeping a journal (and I sure hope you have), your responses to the prompts from the first section will be beneficial for the process you will focus on in this chapter.

Most people, in childhood, were not clearly told that their bodies fell short of some cultural or familial ideal. Instead, they got the message that their body was a problem. They absorbed rules about food and movement, along with beliefs about aging, from tangential comments, non-verbal communication, and intuitive and sensitive observations. For example, I'll never forget a client whose parent always seemed to have something they needed to do in the kitchen while she was having a bedtime snack. She felt she was being supervised or monitored, and her parent disapproved of her eating a snack, but this was never openly discussed.

You may have picked up on messages about bodies and aging, food, and movement because you are more sensitive and intuitive. The good news is that those around you benefit from your sensitivity. Sensitive people have a greater capacity for empathy, so much so that they are more compassionate and are more likely to take action in the face of suffering. If you are sensitive, you are more likely to be creative due to your greater attention to your experience.

The downside of being more sensitive is that you are more likely to feel what others are experiencing and pick up on nonverbal cues. You may need to work on setting boundaries around your tendency to want to care for others. You may also become overstimulated due to increased sensory awareness, requiring managing your exposure to environments and people you find too stimulating.

If you were sensitive as a child, you were likely aware of the emotions and behaviors of others about bodies, aging, food, and movement. For example, you may have noticed:

- The sigh your mother made when you asked for a larger serving of mashed potatoes
- A comment you overheard from the front seat when your grandmother was praising your sibling's thin and athletic body, with no mention of you
- Your mother no longer taking you out for ice cream on Friday afternoons after you no longer fit in your jeans
- When you joined him on bike rides, your mostly absent dad paid more attention to you

- The look of disapproval on your grandfather's face when you returned home after your first year at college
- Your father impatiently shaking his head when your grandmother walked more slowly than the other members of your family
- Feeling left out when your parents and siblings wanted to hike again when they knew hiking wasn't your cup of tea
- Your mother skipping lunch and announcing that she had "forgotten to eat" in a way that felt virtuous
- Your father asking, "Are you sure?" when you asked for another cookie.

You may have interpreted judgments that younger bodies were superior to older bodies; thinner, more athletic bodies were more valued. You learned certain foods were bad or "junk," and others were good or "healthier" choices. You understood gaining weight is just bad, period, no matter what. Therefore, losing weight is always a good thing. These messages were internalized beneath your conscious awareness as a sensitive and intuitive person. You may have also received body shaming, ageist, and diet culture messages that were loud and clear from your family and caregivers, and there was nothing subtle about it.

As Ashton Applewhite says in her must-read book *This Chair Rocks: A Manifesto Against Ageism*, "Nobody's born ageist, but it starts young. Research suggests that children develop negative stereotypes about old age in early childhood, around the same time that attitudes about race and gender begin to form." As you've learned throughout this book, internalized ageism is harmful. Isn't it worth the effort to offer the generations that follow us a perspective laced with a little less ageism?

Is your body image inherited?

When I begin to talk to clients about how their family may have influenced their relationship with their bodies, they will usually say something like, "No, they never made comments about my body." Then they go on to say, "But my mom hated her thighs and talked about them all the time. So when I started gaining weight in puberty, I worried about my thighs getting too big too. I still focus on them. When I try on clothing, I'm always checking to see how my thighs are looking."

A study published (Deek et al., 2023) in *Body Image* found that appearance pressures and fat talk from mothers and sisters are associated with higher levels of body dissatisfaction, dieting or eating restriction, and bulimic behaviors, with mothers having more significant influence. Appearance pressures from mothers and sisters can lead to young women becoming more likely to engage in their own appearance comparisons and internalize beliefs about the thin ideal.

According to a review published by *Common Sense Media* in 2015, children aged 5–8 who think their moms are dissatisfied with their own bodies are likely to have those same ideas about their bodies. Fathers and other family members likely also play a role in body image development but the research is not as common. I'm scratching my head and wondering if this is more about our tendency to blame moms. In my clinical experience, a father's relationship with his body, movement, and food rules are certainly relevant and impactful.

The body dissatisfaction to dieting to disordered eating pipeline likely started at home for you and your parents—and your children and maybe your grandchildren.

Beyond blame: Genetics and disordered eating

While there is no doubt that eating disorders and disordered eating are complex with multiple contributing factors, genetics have been found to play a significant role. Both twin studies and other recent studies have identified specific genetic variants that are associated with an increased risk of eating disorders. These genetic variants are thought to affect brain regulation of eating behavior, body image, and mood, which are all potential contributing factors to eating disorder development.

While a genetic test does not exist yet to predict your vulnerability to developing an eating disorder, the best way to know whether you are genetically at risk is to consider your family history. Consider your relatives and see if they have struggled with disordered eating. If so, you may have a genetic vulnerability and an increased risk, which should make you very wary of diet culture. Remember, you can't know someone has an eating disorder by looking at them.

Intergenerational diet culture, trauma, and epigenetics, oh my!

Intergenerational diet culture involves passing down rules about food, eating, movement, and body image from one generation to the next. Likely, your parents inherited their beliefs about aging, bodies, food, and movement from their parents (your grandparents), which lie well beneath the surface of conscious awareness. Another way to see this is as "legacy burdens."

Many of my clients report first noticing legacy burdens when they return home from family visits. For example, the family story that your maternal grandmother "eats like a bird" and your maternal grandfather makes inappropriate comments about bodies may explain why your mother seems stuck in diet culture and why you are now motivated to read a book like this one so you don't pass the same mess to your children. And If you're thinking "it's too late," repair is possible, keep reading.

I've worked with clients diagnosed with complex PTSD whose caregivers weighed them before mealtimes and provided food based on the number on the scales, withheld food as punishment, or forced them to sit at the table for hours, expecting them to eat everything on their plates despite their dislikes or intolerances. I've had many more clients whose parents ignored their requests for food and rigidly controlled the food environment, or who experienced chaotic food and eating environments. There is a spectrum of severity of intergenerational trauma related to food, eating, movement, and body image. The common outcome is damage to your ability to connect with your body and trust yourself to regulate your eating and movement, along with the possible development of body judgment and criticism and disordered eating.

Intergenerational trauma can also be rooted in historical trauma. Collective trauma and negative community forces, such as racism, oppression, weight stigma, and food insecurity, are all risk factors for eating disorders. Those whose identities are further from the default body are pushed to the margins and are especially vulnerable to trauma, both physically and psychologically, across generations.

I vividly remember the jaw-dropping amazement I experienced when I first learned about epigenetics and its potential relationship to the development of eating disorders. This is a nerdy deep dive, but you will see why understanding the complex nature of intergenerational patterns is essential.

Epigenetics refers to how experiences and environment can cause changes that affect the way your genes work. This research is in its infancy, but for now, experts are connecting cross-generational patterns of eating disorders and investigating whether trauma might be one possible source, among others. For example, if your mother experiences chronic hunger in addition to other trauma for any reason while she is pregnant with you, will this affect you?

Scientists believe that our ancestors' experiences can shift our DNA before we're even born, which might explain one way trauma trickles down through generations and potentially compromises physical and psychological health. In 2011, Rosebloom et al. discovered that those who were conceived during the famine of the "Dutch Hunger Winter" experienced long-term effects on their mental health, including depression and a heightened stress response, as well as impacts on physical health. A 2014 study by Dias and Ressler, shocked mice while sniffing a cherry-like scent, and found that subsequent generations had the same fear associated with the cherry scent despite never being shocked. Even the mice conceived through in-vitro fertilization (via the sperm of a traumatized mouse) were afraid of the cherry scent.

So, the trauma of our parents and grandparents can impact us without us ever directly experiencing or knowing about their trauma. And can our children and grandchildren be affected by our traumatic experiences? You'll learn more about passing intergenerational diet culture, fat phobia, and ageism later on. I encourage you to allow this information to expand your perception of your parents' and grandparents' beliefs and behaviors and those you may have passed down to your children and grandchildren. Please try to drop the blame and shame and offer yourself more compassion and curiosity.

Tender repair: A journey of re-parenting

Now that you can step back and see the complex roots of the beliefs you've inherited about food, eating, movement, body, and aging, I hope it's easier for you to find compassion for those who contributed to damaging diet culture, body shame, and ageism. And while you muster up some compassion for others, please offer some to yourself. As I've said, you will likely get stuck in shame and blame without self-compassion. Self-compassion is essential and comes with practice.

Re-parenting by providing food security, so you do not wait too long to eat and prevent getting too hungry. Repairing damage through re-parenting means seeing food without judgments, so no foods are forbidden, and no foods have superpowers. To do the latter, you will need to dismantle your internalized diet culture thoughts. As you play your parent's role, nourish yourself on a flexible but consistent schedule to feel more secure and experience no sense of scarcity or judgment around food.

Healing from trauma is complex and outside the scope of this book. If what is offered here is not accessible to you, please consider working with a therapist and/or a Registered Dietitian who specializes in eating disorders and trauma.

Body centering and journal prompts

With a base of self-compassion under your feet, step into re-parenting yourself as a way to mend intergenerational diet culture and body shaming. Before you begin, recall your childhood experiences around food, eating, and movement and your body. This can be triggering, so please take good care of yourself, move slowly, and skip this section if you do not feel safe. You may want to consider working through this with the support of a registered dietitian/nutritionist or therapist who specializes in treating eating disorders.

Begin by tuning into your body as you've learned to do. If you feel dysregulated during this journaling exercise, return to your grounding practice. It is helpful to remind yourself that these experiences are in the past and that you are now safe and able to nourish, rest, and move your body as you wish.

As you respond to the following prompts, consider your age when experiencing these events.

- What messages about food, weight, or appearance did you hear from family members growing up?
- Did you believe there were "good" and "bad" foods as a child? How were these food beliefs communicated to you?
- Did family members praise or criticize bodies of family members? How about other people when you were outside your home?

- Was weight, appearance, or fitness a common topic of your family's conversations?
- How did witnessing or participating in these family discussions about dieting, fitness, or weight feel to you?
- Do you remember feeling judged or praised for your body, eating, or movement habits? Do you think of this often?
- What emotions arise when remembering family meals or food-related memories?
- What about when you remember family activities or movement-related memories?
- Did you notice skipping meals, restriction, overeating, or dieting patterns in your family?
- Did you notice activity and movement patterns in your family?
- Do you remember specific moments when you resisted or embraced the norms of diet culture in your family? What prompted these choices? How did your family respond?
- What would you say to the part of yourself that experienced diet culture in childhood if you wrote a letter to your younger self about food, movement, and body image?

Now that you have a clearer picture of your experiences in childhood let's consider what it might look like to approach nourishing and moving your body free of diet culture. *It is never too late and you are never too old to heal this damage.*

Another way to approach nourishing your (younger) self

In my long career as a Registered Dietitian specializing in preventing and treating disordered eating, and as a parent and grandparent, I learned to trust two evidence-based approaches to nourishing children: the Division of Responsibility (DOR) developed by Evelyn Satter, MS, RD, LCSW, and the Responsive

Feeding Approach. My adult clients find these approaches beneficial as a framework to support re-parenting themselves around
eating and movement. I offer these to you as powerful tools for
healing the damage of intergenerational diet culture.

Division of Responsibility (DOR)

Like most new mothers, I was on a quest to read all the things
before I had my first child in 1989. One of those books was
Ellyn Satter's *Child of Mine: Feeding with Love and Good Sense*.
I was hooked. I read the rest of her books and soon utilized her
Division of Responsibility with clients when appropriate. The
DOR goes like this:

Parents are responsible for the following:

- What foods are brought into the home, encouraging a variety of foods with no food hierarchy, all are valued
- When foods are eaten with a flexible and consistent schedule
- Where foods are eaten with a flexible preference being at the
  family table.

Children are responsible for:

- What and how much they choose to eat.

Responsive Feeding (RF) approach

Responsive eating is a "reciprocal process between a parent and
an infant where infants communicate their hunger and fullness
cues, and parents respond to these cues," according to Black and
Aboud in their 2011 article. Responsive feeding is embedded in
a theoretical framework of responsive parenting. This process is
a dance between the child and caregiver that fosters the child's
autonomy and self-regulation, honoring the child's hunger and
fullness cues.

The child initiates the beginning and end of feeding by
expressing hunger and fullness both verbally and non-verbally.
The caregiver promptly responds to the child's signals with

emotional support. Children who experience these predictable responses develop trust in themselves and their caregivers, a sense of security, and a capacity to self-regulate.

This division encourages parents to allow the child to discover their food preferences and how much food their bodies need to feel satisfied. The goal is for the child to develop autonomy and trust in their body's ability to regulate while the parents exhibit trust in their child's body and competency. The Responsive Feeding Approach is very similar, with less structure than DOR.

Imagine if you'd been offered autonomy as a child and learned to trust your body! The good news is that it is not too late to repair any harm by re-parenting yourself with this system. If you've tried "Intuitive Eating," you may notice some similarities.

Get curious and playful as the younger parts of yourself explore and try to tune in to notice what foods make you feel good, what foods are satisfying, what foods you enjoy, and what foods leave you feeling unwell or tired. Have fun! Be aware, you may not start out trusting yourself and may feel resistant to this idea.

Ultimately, the goal is to learn to trust yourself and your body. As discussed in Chapter 5, this can take some time and does not follow a linear path. You will have easier days and more challenging days. But the freedom and empowerment available to you are life-changing if you choose this process!

Internal Family Systems (IFS) and intergenerational diet culture

Internal Family Systems (IFS) can help to understand the damage of intergenerational diet culture and heal this damage. IFS was developed in the 1980s by psychologist Richard Schwartz, PhD and has gained popularity in the field of eating disorder treatment. Schwartz's clients described their inner lives as "Parts," which he defined as "conflicted subpersonalities that reside within them." Generally, these Parts evolve to assist us in navigating life, especially as a response to difficult or overwhelming situations. These components are natural and universal aspects of the mind, often formed to fulfill specific roles or provide protection.

There are three primary components of the internal family system:

- Core Self
- Wounded Parts
- Protective Parts.

Each possesses subpersonalities with distinct functions. The IFS model helps Parts shift to more adaptive roles while elevating the Core Self to lead the system, fostering balance and harmony.

There are no "bad" Parts, which is the title of one of Schwartz's recent books. Life experiences—such as trauma—can foster unhealthy roles, leading to disorganization within the system. For instance, when a child witnesses their mother criticizing her own body, the child might form a Part aimed at protecting them from feeling unlovable due to having a similar body type. Consequently, that Part may restrict food intake or over-exercise. This can create confusion since such actions can be harmful; however, the Part enforcing this diet culture believes it shields you from criticism and rejection.

Protective Parts shield you from emotional distress, harm, or vulnerability. For instance, a "manager" Part may develop to keep you safe by increasing controlling behaviors or avoiding risks. Suppose you witnessed your father criticizing larger bodies. In that case, a Part of you may have developed patterns of restriction or over-exercising to keep you within the thin ideal, therefore protecting you from the possibility of your body also receiving criticism.

"Exiles" are Parts that carry painful memories, emotions, or experiences that your internal system keeps hidden to protect you from the pain associated with re-experiencing hurt or trauma. Keeping yourself hungry or under the weight your body is genetically designed to weigh, over-exercising, or eating past the point of fullness can all serve to "numb" you or be a way that you've learned to zone out or dissociate.

When you experienced trauma or significant emotional distress earlier in your life, Parts may have formed as coping mechanisms. These Parts bear the burden of trauma (exiles) or strive to prevent you re-experiencing it (managers). If you are a "pleaser," this Part of you may have developed to seek approval or distraction when there was a conflict in your family. A "critic" Part of you might have emerged to drive you toward success in a demanding environment if you thought your success meant a sense of belonging, worthiness, or even love.

You can see how it is understandable that the legacy burden from intergenerational diet culture and fat phobia created pleaser and critic Parts of you. The "pleaser" Part of you now emerges as body shaming thoughts if you have a friend who is talking about how someone has "let themselves go" when they are no longer chronically dieting. Or the "critic" Part emerges as guilt and anxiety about your eating behavior over a holiday.

Parts help you function and survive in an unpredictable or unsafe world. Each Part serves a unique purpose, such as ensuring you adhere to societal or familial norms or helping you to cope with challenging emotions. If you perceive that you must look younger to be loved by a partner or belong to a group, your Parts will protect you from rejection and abandonment by encouraging more choices that align with an anti-aging or diet-culture mindset.

In more complicated instances, Parts arise to manage your internal conflicts. For example, one Part may urge risk-taking, like starting an aggressive diet program or drug, while another may seek to inhibit it. This polarization often mirrors competing needs or fears within your internal system.

When the Self (your core, compassionate, wise center) has been diminished by trauma, including the trauma of chronic dieting or disordered eating, some Parts become "burdened" and assume extreme roles or beliefs. They take over in the void left by the Self and assume protective measures that may not serve your best interests. For instance, if you've experienced criticism or neglect, a Part of you might carry the story "I am not good enough." If a Part of you feels you are not worthy of effort and attention, then diet culture, disordered eating, and anti-aging messages join in, adding to the feeling that you are never enough and you are never doing enough.

The "Self" is intended to play a leading role within your internal system.

According to IFS, qualities of the Self consist of the 8Cs and 5Ps:

- 8Cs: connectedness, confidence, compassion, calmness, creativity, courage, clarity, and compassion

- 5Ps: presence, playfulness, patience, persistence, and perspective.

The IFS process assists your Parts in unburdening, re-establishing their connection with the Self, and returning to their natural, balanced functions. This process promotes harmony and healing within your internal system, enabling each Part to feel recognized, valued, and supported.

An essential aspect of IFS is differentiating protective and wounded Parts. This empowers your Self to reclaim leadership by reconnecting with your C and P qualities. First, understand different aspects of yourself, then recognize how they influence your thoughts and behaviors, and, lastly, process trauma and painful experiences to alleviate your burdens. The unburdening process takes place in these six essential steps or 6Fs of the IFS model:

1 *Find*: First, identify when and where you feel certain Parts getting activated—including where it is in the body. Which Part seems to need your attention? Getting curious about

these experiences may be supported through meditation, mindfulness, or paying attention to bodily sensations. The body check-ins you've practiced throughout this book are a powerful way to scan your body for these sensations.

2 *Focus*: Prompt self-reflection about the Parts you identified in the step above. Focus on each Part and tune into it individually, paying attention to how it makes you feel. Using art instead of words may help you connect with your Parts. Watercolor was extremely helpful for me when I began my IFS journey. My first painting was a meeting place for my Self and my Parts, which was a beautiful, expansive, calm horizon.

3 *Flesh out*: Define your Parts and learn more about each of them. For example, ask how the Part looks. Then, describe how you feel when you are connected to this Part of yourself and your proximity to it. This can be a journal entry, a quick note to yourself, or even an art project.

4 *Feeling*: In this step, define how you feel toward protective Parts vs the self. How does this Part influence your thoughts and behaviors in general and, more specifically, about eating, movement, and your body? For example, are you ashamed, surprised, sad, angry, or annoyed by a perfectionist Part of you and the role it assumes? How do you feel about your behaviors, attitudes, thoughts, and reactions associated with your perfectionism? Noting how many of the 8Cs or Core Self is present is crucial in determining whether the wounded or protective Part is in charge. It can be helpful to journal, draw, or paint about this.

5 *Befriend*: Next, get to know the Part and learn more about the Part you're focusing on. Then, begin to befriend this Part of yourself as best you can. If you are angry with this Part, for example, perhaps your perfectionism has been a Part of your disordered eating, and you do not appreciate the way you've felt pressured to be perfect. It may help to remember this Part has been trying to protect you from perceived harm. You

may be curious about how this Part of you was developed in the first place, and try to find out what it needs. It may seem strange to talk to yourself this way, but you already speak to yourself to some degree. This is a helpful and healing conversation with Parts of yourself.

6 *Fear*: This final step is about understanding what the Part fears and what it protects you from. You might want to ask the Part about its goal and what would happen if it wasn't in charge. Another way to think about this is that you may no longer need this Part to protect you and may need to be updated to your current situation. For example, you may want to be more flexible with your food choices and no longer feel the need to eat "perfectly," so you may need to connect with the perfectionist Part to thank them for trying to protect you from judgment and criticism, and you no longer feel the need to be "perfect."

The Resources section includes several places to learn more about IFS. At any point in your healing process, you may want to seek the support of a therapist or Registered Dietitian who specializes in and eating disorder treatment.

Now that you've learned more about how you've inherited diet culture and body shame, how this has affected you and your relationship with your body and others, and how you can heal from these belief systems, do you think you also passed diet culture, anti-fat bias, and ageism along to the next generation?

Healing damage to your children and grandchildren

As we've discussed, you may have been exposing others, like your children and grandchildren, to harmful thoughts and beliefs before you understood the potential damage of diet culture, ageism, and body shame. You may not have recognized the water you were swimming in as damaging to you. Therefore, you may have invited others to join you in going for a swim, thinking the water was fine. Please give yourself grace here. You can't do better until you know better.

Diet culture, disordered eating, and over-exercising are normalized, sometimes even praised, in our culture. Let that sink in. Due to this normalization, one of the biggest challenges is recognizing diet culture and disordered eating in and around you and seeing it for what it is.

Here's a refresher.

Diet culture is a system of beliefs inherited from your family and culture that prioritizes weight, shape, and size over well-being. It equates thinness and specific body types with health, morality, and success while promoting restrictive eating, excessive exercise, and the pursuit of an "ideal" body. Diet culture is perpetuated through media, marketing, medical advice, and cultural norms, often disguising itself as "health" or "wellness."

Key features of diet culture:

- *Thin idealization*: Establishes thinness as the benchmark for beauty and health, suggesting that staying thin helps us stay relevant as we age.
- *Food morality*: Categorizes foods as "good" or "bad," leading to feelings of guilt and shame associated with eating.
- *Disconnecting from and distrusting the body*: Guidelines for eating and exercise are derived from external sources or so-called "experts," who ignore our internal signals and intuition.
- *Weight stigma*: Marginalizes those with larger bodies and perpetuates the belief that health is solely determined by weight.
- *Overemphasis on control*: Encourages the idea that controlling one's weight or size is a personal responsibility and moral imperative.

When you love a child, you want the very best for them. In a fat-phobic world, you are likely well-intentioned in offering guidance for a child's eating and movement to control their body size and shape as a way to protect them (just like your protective parts show up with more diet culture advice for you).

But we know children benefit significantly from living in a home free from diet culture, food rules, weight stigma, and fat phobia. A home where children learn that their bodies are loved unconditionally and can be trusted is far more protective than exposure to diet culture, which is damaging.

Just to be clear, here are the primary reasons diet/ wellness culture is harmful to you, your children, and your grandchildren:

- *Promotes disordered eating*: Following someone else's rules about nourishing your body encourages you to override and ignore your body's cues and instincts, which is the root of disordered eating. Unhealthy behaviors include food restriction, binge eating, or compulsive exercise. Chronic dieting leads to weight cycling, which is well documented as negatively impacting physical and mental health.
- *Damages body image and causes devastating body shame*: Diet culture creates unrealistic standards of beauty and health, fostering comparison and feelings of inadequacy, shame, and self-hatred. What happens when your body resembles the "before" picture of the "before and after" testimonials of diet culture? Diet culture promotes the idea that your self-worth is tied to your body size, shape, and appearance.
- *Neglects true health*: One of the most confusing aspects of diet culture is that it centers on your weight rather than your true well-being, ignoring significant aspects of health, such as mental health and social connections. The shadow side of wellness culture is that it can mask eating disorders or other health problems under the guise of "clean eating" or "fitness."
- *Perpetuates weight stigma*: Discriminates against people in larger bodies, leading to social, medical, and professional

bias. Research shows that experiencing weight stigma impacts your physical and mental health and contributes to shame and isolation. Isolation and loneliness contribute to poor physical and mental health, especially as you age.

Throughout this book, I've encouraged you to challenge the body hierarchy and narrative you've inherited and which still surrounds you about your body and how you "should" nourish and move it. Now, I am asking you to also reflect on the biases you hold about bodies, especially the bodies of your loved ones. Once you understand that diet culture and ageism is damaging to your children and grandchildren, I'm sure you do not want to be another source of these harmful messages. But what if you have already passed this mess down to the next generations before you became aware?

Apologies and repair

Before we step into the work of repair, please give yourself some **significant** self-compassion. We've established that you inherited your ageism, body hierarchy, diet culture beliefs, and disordered eating thoughts and behaviors. Your children and grandchildren may have simply witnessed these parts of you. You may have encouraged them to join you in these beliefs and behaviors, thinking that was in their best interest. You potentially unknowingly caused harm. **So now that you know better, you can do better.**

Again, no shame. No blame. Only continuing to learn and grow.

Repairing the damage caused by passing diet culture, ageism, and disordered eating to the next generation involves honest, vulnerable, and open dialogue. This is not easy. I encourage my clients to write what they want to say, which they may or may not actually send to their loved ones. This offers a way for you to gain some clarity on what you would like to say, or it could serve as a statement you would like to send before a conversation takes place. Here are some essential steps in this healing process.

1. Acknowledge and take responsibility

See the impact: First, you must accept that perpetuating ageism and diet culture, even unintentionally, can affect younger generations' relationships with food, movement, body image, their perception of aging, and self-worth.

Apologize for real: Explain your journey, what you are learning, and how you are changing, and acknowledge how your beliefs or actions might have affected them. A genuine apology to your children and grandchildren who have been impacted by your ageism, disordered eating or diet culture beliefs and behaviors can be powerful.

Nobody teaches us how to apologize, even though apologies are essential for healthy relationships. So, I want to briefly mention the components of a genuine apology based on the incredible work of Harriet Lerner, Ph.D., which can be found in her book, *Why Won't You Apologize? Healing Big Betrayals and Everyday Hurts*.

According to Lerner:

> "A good apology is an opportunity for us to take clear and direct responsibility for our wrongdoing without evading, blaming, making excuses, or dredging up offenses from the past. It brims with accountability, meets the moment, and can transform our relationships."

Sounds pretty important, right? Here are six essentials of a genuine apology:

- *Drop your defenses*: Keep an open mind and listen to understand the other party with the same degree of passion of being understood.

- *Be genuine*: When apologizing for something, it's critical to show genuine remorse and vulnerability, letting go of being in control of the situation and the outcome.
- *No qualifiers*: A sincere apology does not include caveats or qualifiers. "'But' almost always signifies a rationalization, a criticism, or an excuse," Lerner says. "It doesn't matter if what you say after the 'but' is true, the 'but' makes your apology false."
- *Be calm and succinct*: Keep your apology brief and free of drama. Showing up as the one who needs emotional support centers you and not the person you are apologizing to.
- *Stay focused*: Zero in on the situation at hand and stay attuned to the needs of the hurting person. True healing takes place when the person feels seen and understood and that you genuinely care. "I'm sorry" can feel meaningless if genuine care and understanding are missing.
- *The beginning*: A well-done apology can be an opening created in a relationship. It may be an opportunity to repair damage and to strengthen and deepen a relationship. You'll find more about apologies in the Resources section.

2. Pass down what you've learned

Offer to share what you've learned about the harm of ageism, diet culture, and disordered eating with your children and grandchildren, along with the benefits of adopting an age-affirming and anti-ageist, non-restrictive, weight and food-neutral approach to nourishing and caring for your body. The Resources section is an excellent source to share.

3. Model a healthier relationship with food, movement, and your body relationship

Dismantle food rules: By modeling healthier behaviors, you can show your children and grandchildren that foods are not inherently "good" or "bad."

Decenter appearance and drop body shame: Talk about your body more neutrally, maybe even with acceptance and celebration. Avoid criticizing and judging all bodies, including your own. Celebrate yourself and others without focusing on appearance. Here are a few examples, and you can find an expansive list on my website at DebraBenfield.com.

- Your eyes are full of energy today. You are positively glowing.
- You have such a kind heart. I feel much better when I see you.
- It just makes me so happy to see you.
- Seeing you reminds me of how lucky I am.
- Seeing you is one of my favorite things.
- I'm so happy to see you and can't wait to _______.

4. Encourage critical thinking

Challenge cultural norms: Have conversations with your children and grandchildren that question societal messages about beauty, weight, aging, and appearance as they relate to worth. Point out unrealistic and ridiculous standards in media and advertising.

Discuss media literacy: Help your children and grandchildren to recognize and reject ageism and manipulative diet culture messages in social and other media.

5. Invite open communication

Create a safe space: Encourage your children and grandchildren to share their feelings about food, body image, ageism, and societal pressures without fear of judgment.

Listen actively: Be curious and validate their experiences and emotions. Notice if you are dismissive or minimizing their struggles and process that. It may mean it's time for another genuine apology.

6. Promote self-acceptance and body neutrality

Focus on bodies as our homes and life partners: Emphasize that our bodies support our ability to live and experience our lives, including pleasure, rather than valuing ourselves based on our appearance.

Celebrate diversity: Talk about how bodies come in all shapes, sizes, ages, and abilities and are worthy of respect and care.

7. Advocate for change

When you are able, speak up when you notice weight stigma, ageism, and diet culture in other relationships, your community, schools, and online spaces. Treat weight stigma and ageism just as you would when you notice racism or other systems of oppression.

8. Be patient with yourself and the process

Dismantling internalized ageism, diet culture, and weight stigma and repairing the damage they cause will take time. Mistakes may happen, but your consistency and commitment to change can help heal and create a legacy of body liberation.

9. Don't hesitate to seek professional support if you need help

Family therapy: Consider working with a therapist specializing in disordered eating and family dynamics to repair relationships and unlearn harmful patterns together.

Registered dietitians and therapists: Work with weight-neutral professionals to foster a positive relationship between food and health.

> **Naomi's story**
> Naomi was among the first to sign up for my group coaching program several years ago. She was 64 years old and had a kind and quiet disposition. During our group sessions, she tended to be concerned about everyone having a chance to speak and wanted to ensure she was not taking "too much of our time."

Growing up, both of Naomi's parents commented on her body, starting at age 10, based on her memories, and continuing through high school and college. They also made comments judging other people's bodies to one another, along with expressing plenty of opinions about their own bodies.

Her parents' had semi-constant conversations about their diet and exercise programs. Foods like chips and cookies were considered "junk" food and rarely brought into her home.

When she saw her grandparents, they would criticize her parents' bodies and, to a lesser extent, her body, and give her confusing messages about food. They would take Naomi to bakeries or ice cream shops, which she loved, but in the next breath tell her to keep this a secret from her parents. At dinner, they would ask her, "Are you sure you really need that?" when Naomi would ask for seconds.

As a sensitive and intuitive little girl, she worried about her body and compared herself to other little girls as early as elementary school. Ultimately, she described herself as a child and teenager as "self-conscious" about her body and appearance, wanting to cover herself with layers and loose clothing.

Naomi remembered starting to sneak food as a young child. When she began visiting friends, she would be overjoyed to see cookie jars and snack drawers at their houses. Sometimes, she would sneak down to their kitchens at night when everyone was asleep to have more of these special treats.

By the time Naomi was in high school, she was engaging in cycles of restricting and binge eating with movement following the same "all or nothing" pattern. She started experimenting with laxatives as a way to "get rid of "the food she'd eaten and realized that her mom did the same thing. Naomi also joined her dad in going for a run to "get rid of" the food she felt guilty about eating, and sometimes she would purge through vomiting. These patterns became more consistent in college, where she found a roommate and sorority sisters with similar behaviors.

Naomi met her husband in college. He continued the job her parents started, openly commenting on her eating, encouraging her to "work out," and even monitoring her weight, except when she was pregnant. So, during her pregnancies, she loved the freedom from surveillance. She felt like she was eating to "make up for lost time" and stopped her bulimic behaviors. She was pregnant three times and would return to her diet and exercise regime as soon as she delivered her babies.

Then, Naomi's husband started commenting on how she fed their children, how they ate, and about their bodies. Naomi felt guilty that she did not push back and she was passing down the systems of diet culture to her children. They witnessed her dieting and body-shaming comments and experienced their own strict food and exercise rules growing up. When Naomi joined the group, she talked about witnessing her children doing the same to her grandchildren, which broke her heart. This was what made her want to join our group but part of her wondered if it was too late or if she was too old to change.

Naomi and her husband divorced when their last child left for college. Naomi had been in and out of therapy since she was a teenager but had not discussed her disordered eating and body shame. More recently, she started focusing on these issues in therapy and also joined my group coaching program for more support and community. Like so many people who join my group, Naomi felt very isolated and like she was "the only one" wanting to opt out of anti-aging and diet culture and break the legacy burden of body shame.

When we started discussing intergenerational trauma, Naomi shared that her Jewish ancestry included family members surviving the holocaust. There was a big "aha" moment for her when we examined the relationship between epigenetics, trauma, and disordered eating. She found herself more compassionate toward others and herself when she developed a greater understanding of the roots of the disordered eating and body shame she inherited.

During her time with our group program, Naomi shared her body liberation journey with her children to repair the damage she felt she had contributed to. She started by apologizing to each of them and committed to protecting her grandchildren from the same damaging messages. Through it all, Naomi was incredibly vulnerable with our group, which empowered her to do the same with her children. She was exceptionally courageous and fiercely devoted to passing down body liberation rather than more of the ageism, body shame, and diet culture mess. I get goosebumps just remembering Naomi's story! She decided that she was willing to do what she could to heal her relationship with her body, do her best to repair the damage with her kids, and hopefully protect her grandkids. Not all heroes wear capes, indeed!

It didn't start with you, but it can end with you—body liberation as your legacy

Body liberation is a movement rooted in the belief that you and all of us are free to live in our bodies just as we are. Body liberation is an absolutely radical concept in today's youth and thin obsessed culture. It defies societal and familial expectations around size, shape, age, and appearance. Embracing it means recognizing that your body—and all bodies—are inherently worthy of respect, love, and acceptance, regardless of age, size, shape, appearance, race, ability or health status.

As we've discussed, diet culture, body shame, ageism, weight stigma, anti-fat bias, and fat phobia are your legacy burdens. When you are able to break free from these burdens and limiting belief systems, your body is the cauldron of the transformation, the source of the alchemy that shifts your legacy from burden to body liberation. This radical change is not linear, easy, or fast. This life-giving process is messy, prone to fits and starts, brings good days and bad days, and takes time. I talked to some experts about what this might require and look like in your life.

Virginia Sole-Smith's *Fat Talk: Parenting in the Age of Diet Culture* is a must-read to protect a child you love or your inner child from diet culture. In her final chapter, she lists eight actions, or "Fat Talks," where you can challenge the fat phobia and diet culture in your world. Number Three is "How to talk to your mother (and father, and every Baby Boomer)," so I contacted Ms. Sole-Smith to talk more about this meaningful conversation.

When I asked Virginia how grandparents can help stop intergenerational diet culture and body shame, she said she has:

> "compassion for the vulnerability that may arise for grandparents as their roles have shifted. They no longer have control or may regret how they parented their kids at this age. But it's not the role of a grandparent to editorialize about food and body choices unless advice has been sought out."

Instead, respect boundaries when interjecting with your advice or judging food choices and eating. Ask yourself, "How do I enter this with love?" When considering how you interact with your kids and grandkids about food, Virginia recommends asking yourself questions like:

- How can we connect over food?
- How can food be something we find mutual pleasure in?
- Can we create a sweet tradition around food?
- How can food be something that will ground our relationship?

Notes from an expert

While it is in everyone's best interest, including yours, for your kids and grandkids to witness your modeling a comfortable relationship with eating, movement, and your body, that's a tall order! While you are working toward that, start by no longer sharing thoughts reflecting your body and food fears and worries. Ms. Sole-Smith remarks:

> "No longer narrating your struggle is a kindness to yourself and those around you. Start by trying not to speak about how we perform, punishing ourselves and atoning for our bodies. For example, you don't have to make pejorative statements about your body when you put on a swimsuit. You don't have to talk about needing to go for a walk after eating your Thanksgiving meal. That's a script that we can outright say I won't do that anymore. When I verbalize it, I'm teaching and modeling to my kids and grandkids that this is the right way to think about this stuff and I don't want to do that anymore."

I was also fortunate to interview Oona Hanson, a nationally recognized writer, educator, and parent coach who supports families in navigating diet culture and eating disorders. Hanson is also the author of the much-loved Substack newsletter *Parenting Without Diet Culture.*

Notes from an expert

Oona offered wise advice, reminding us that "we cannot dismantle diet culture in ourselves and those we love using the tools of diet culture, such as perfectionism, black-and-white thinking, rigidity, and shame." Rather, prioritize the health of the relationship and connection and approach this communication with compassion as we consider the larger context of vast changes in recommendations for how we parent and feed our children.

Oona reminds us:

> "No one is harming kids intentionally, but our words matter. Joking and teasing done in the spirit of love with no ill intent can still do harm. We don't know which comments about bodies, eating, and exercise will stick and haunt a child, including comments parents and grandparents make about their own bodies."

She warns that "diet culture is so strong. Our indoctrination in it is so deep that parents and grandparents may not recognize the harm of their comments even after a child has been hospitalized to treat a deadly eating disorder." I have seen the same phenomenon in my clinical practice.

Whatever the circumstances, Oona encourages us to talk to those we love about the harm of diet culture and body shame.

> "There can be so much healing when this conversation takes place with compassion. There can be collective acknowledgment of the harm done and maybe even experience grief when you realize that you've spent so much time and energy caught up in diet culture. Maybe you didn't even know there was another way."

This brings to mind that lovely Maya Angelou quote:

> "Do the best you can until you know better. Then, when you know better, do better."

I know you've been doing the best you can. Now, you know better so you can do better.

You are worthy of the effort to liberate yourself from the burdens of body criticism, ageism, and diet culture. And it is also true that sometimes, witnessing the burden in your loved ones may motivate you to do this work. You and those around you will benefit from your labor.

You may remember my discussion of "relational ageism" and the research of Tracey Gendron, Ph.D., that I discussed in the first chapter. During my interview with her about her research, she ended our conversation with some inspiring words:

> "The fact remains that tiny little changes make a difference: one person, one interaction at a time. With tools to interrupt ageism, we can think about our aging bodies differently and see ourselves differently, leading to more significant societal change.
>
> Narratives change. To see things differently, people decide to do things differently. That is empowering."

During my interview with Meg Bradbury, body trust coach and program coordinator, who identifies as lesbian/genderqueer, who was in her 60s at the time of this writing, I so resonated with and appreciated their words about the potential for liberation during this season of our lives. They said:

> "What are we holding onto? We want to be seen as human, beloved and have a sense of belonging, especially as we get old. Our community is everything. If there is ever a time that you can let go of the status quo, of the expectations of patriarchal oppression, it is this time in our lives. When I can quiet that noise, this is the most liberating and energizing time of my life. When I can be free from so much bullshit and able to concentrate on myself, where I am, and how I want to be in the world. At this point in my life, freedom can come with being this age without having to mother or parent in an expansive, not biological way. We don't get to explore that because we are kept down and stressed and managed. The word oppression just keeps coming back up because being older in our world is a crime, and we fucking didn't do anything."

In a world where you are bombarded with messages that your body must be a project, to be comfortable in your body just as you are is revolutionary! As Cathi Rae says in this excerpt from her poem, "Mirror Image", published in *Your Cleaner Hates You*:

> This body is its own revolution
> a micro manifesto of change
> I stare into the camera unashamedly myself
> the ghosts of other women line up behind my shoulders

> *Cathi Rae from her poem "Mirror Image,"*
> *published in Your Cleaner Hates You*

My greatest hope is that, after reading this book, you have the tools to interrupt and break free from ageism, body shame, and diet culture. My greatest wish is to that you feel more comfortable and confident about taking up space, especially in this season of your life. *You deserve the pleasure, ease, and freedom to age unapologetically, just as you are in your body in this present moment.*

I created an Aging Unapologetically Manifesto that summarizes the pieces and parts of this journey for you. May this be your North Star.

Conclusion and a manifesto

As you close *Unapologetic Aging*, I invite you to imagine yourself standing before a mirror, a gentle smile playing on your lips.

Some days, you may still avoid the mirror. Other days, you might glance at your reflection and feel a quiet acceptance—"Yep, this is me. Cool." And on some days, you may feel a warm glow rising from your heart, spreading through your body, rooted in the deep knowing that your body is your life partner.

In my mind's eye, you see that your body has softened—and that softening reflects the gentleness you now offer yourself. You're no longer chasing the hardness of body or spirit. You're far less inclined to be hard on yourself.

I invite you to help create a world where bodies that wrinkle, dimple, soften, spot, and wobble are seen with affection and treated with care. Let us celebrate all bodies.

One of my favorite phrases is: "All bodies are worthy bodies." Because it's not just a slogan—it's the truth.

Aging Unapologetically: A Manifesto

1 *I commit to recognizing and dismantling ageism—in myself and in the world.*

I will cultivate awareness of how ageism shows up in my thoughts, language, and actions. I will challenge the ageist beliefs I've internalized and choose to speak to myself in ways that honor my full humanity—not my age. When I encounter ageism in the world around me, I will speak up, knowing that every voice matters in shifting the narative and creating lasting change.

2 *I commit to embracing midlife and beyond with acceptance and affirmation.*

I will meet this new chapter with curiosity, respect, and celebration and when I feel afraid. I will acknowledge and accept my fear, knowing it will pass. I choose to see aging not as a decline, but as a rich and worthy part of my life—full of growth, wisdom, and possibility.

3 *I commit to challenging our culture's body hierarchy and honoring the worth of all bodies.*

I will recognize the ways I've internalized harmful messages about which bodies are deemed more valuable. I commit to unlearning these beliefs and embracing the truth that all bodies—of every size, shape, race, age, ability, sexual orientation, and gender identity—are inherently worthy. There is no wrong way to have a body.

4 *I commit to de-centering my weight in my pursuit of well-being and dismantling diet culture.*

I will question the beliefs I've inherited from diet culture and actively work to dismantle them. I commit to releasing the rigid rules, shame, and moral judgment that diet and fitness culture have imposed on my relationship with food and movement. As

I free myself from these constraints, I will nourish my body with connection, curiosity, and compassion. I will care for myself and include satisfaction and pleasure—choosing a weight-neutral path to well-being.

5 *I commit to cultivating compassionate curiosity through mindful awareness in my daily life to support my well-being.*

I will engage in practices that strengthen my connection to mind, body, and spirit, and deepen my capacity for compassion, curiosity, and acceptance—including self-compassion.

6 *I commit to creating playful and embodied movement to support my well-being.*

I will free myself from the rigidity, guilt, and shame rooted in anti-aging and fitness culture. Instead, I will allow myself to explore how I want to feel in my body—with curiosity, playfulness, and joy.

7 *I commit to practices that support healthy nervous system regulation, rest, and sleep.*

I will deepen my understanding of how I experience dysregulation and learn practices to bring stability and regulation to my nervous system. I will give myself permission to rest and prioritize my sleep health.

8 *I commit to encouraging a more comfortable relationship with my body, body image, and embodied intimacy, honoring bodily autonomy and knowing it's okay to opt out of sexual intimacy, too. My body, my choice.*

Expanding my ability to see the beauty around and within me is softening my judgment and criticism of my body and the bodies of others. As I feel more ease and connection with my body and see my body through a more neutral and accepting lens,

I am also more open to experiencing embodied intimacy in this season of my life.

9 *I commit to engaging in inclusive social connection and activism to support an interdependent community—for myself and others.*

As I expand my understanding of the importance of interconnection and belonging, I will strive to be inclusive and speak up for myself and others in the face of ageism, anti-fat bias, and other forms of oppression. I am becoming more aware of the potential harm in valuing individualism over the collective and community and the wisdom of interdependence.

10 *I commit to making body liberation part of my life's legacy.*

I recognize that many of the limiting beliefs I hold about my aging body were inherited—and I will question and work to unlearn these beliefs. As I heal what was passed down to me, I will also do my best to repair any harm I may have unknowingly passed on to those I love. I choose to leave a legacy rooted in body liberation.

Long Song of My Body

Jillian Hanson

Allow me. I am a multitude within
the same outline. A collapsible tin cup
made for travel, I fold and unfold from
this to this. I am a long song of comfort
and function, a continuous moment
embroidered with many breaths. I am
a sod-house wired with spirits. Watch
as I soften and expand to hold the widening
field of light within. Many selves here,
more and more.

> *One collects stones at the open mouth of Lake Superior.*
> *One chokes on her words in front of her mother.*
> *One cuts class to smoke by the river.*
> *One takes the city bus to theater class.*
> *One stands forsaken at the mirror in cut-off shorts.*
> *One lies to her boyfriend about the rent.*
> *One gets married in a 60-dollar dress.*
> *One labors like a freight train.*
> *One drives carpool, backseat filled with tissue-paper flowers.*

The girls-only film strip in sixth grade
got it wrong. Nothing about being female
resembles those prim line drawings. Not
the rosy hot froth of 400 periods,
nor the petal-pink daughter, blue on arrival.
Not the swell of tonsil, nor the sacrificed
appendix. Purple surgery scars writhe
the skin like worms. Etch runes of protection.

> *One is white-hands-deep in dough.*
> *One pays a visit to divorce court.*
> *One hides a lapful of words at midnight.*
> *One hangs swagger from her hips like a belt.*
> *One teeters on water, patient and wide as lily pads*

You think I am now irrelevant,
uninhabitable. You look away.
But I am not empty. I am a dark jar full.
I keep my blood now, use it for ink.
I cast votes with it. Measure it out
as medicine. Burn it for fuel, hot air
for the balloon.

Watch me rise, good and slow.

Notes and sources

This book is the culmination of my 40-year career as an RD specializing in preventing and treating eating disorders and my more recent research and practice focusing on nutrition, movement, body image, and well-being in midlife and beyond. I created a group coaching program in 2022 and a membership in 2023. Writing this book also draws from the research for my group coaching program and my experience with my extraordinary clients. The material contributing to my perspective and approach to care, in addition to quotes, statistics, and research references throughout this book is listed chapter by chapter below.

Chapter 1

Applewhite, A. (2020) *This Chair Rocks: A Manifesto Against Ageism,* Celadon Books.

Bajekal, Nitu (2024) *Finding Me in Menopause,* Sheldon Press.

Blanchflower, D.G. (2021) "Is happiness U-shaped everywhere? Age and subjective well-being in 145 countries," *J Popul Econ.,* 34(2), 575–624. doi: 10.1007/s00148-020-00797-z. Epub 2020 Sep 9. PMID: 32929308; PMCID: PMC7480662.

Dujmovic, J. (2024) "Billionaires are spending big on anti-aging drugs so they—and maybe you—can live forever," *Market Watch,* August 24. https://www.marketwatch.com/story/billionaires-are-spending-big-so-they-and-maybe-you-can-live-forever-82041ed7#

Galambos, N.L., Krahn, H.J., Johnson, M.D., & Lachman, M.E. (2020) "The U-shape of happiness across the life course: Expanding the discussion," *Perspectives on Psychological Science: A Journal of the Association for Psychological Science,* 15(4), 898. doi: 10.1177/1745691620902428

Gendron, T. (2022) *Ageism Unmasked: Exploring Age Bias and How to End It,* Steerforth Press.

Global Wellness Institute (2024) "Wellness Economy Statistics & Facts," November, https://globalwellnessinstitute.org/press-room/statistics-and-facts/#:~:text=We%20project%20that%20the%20global,in%20 2024%2C%20and%20march%20toward

Levy B.R., Slade M.D., Kunkel S.R., & Kasl S.V. (2002) "Longevity increased by positive self-perceptions of aging," *J Pers Soc Psychol.,* 83(2), 261–70. doi: 10.1037//0022-3514.83.2.261. PMID: 12150226.

Levy, R. (2023) *Breaking the Age Code: How Your Beliefs About Aging Determine How Long and Well You Live*, William Morrow Paperbacks.

Ogihara, Y. & Uchida, Y. (2014) "Does individualism bring happiness? Negative effects of individualism on interpersonal relationships and happiness," *Frontiers in Psychology*, 5, 135. doi: 10.3389/fpsyg.2014.00135

Taylor, Sonya Renee (2021) *The BodyIs Not An Apology: The Power of Radical Self-Love*, Berrett-Koehler Publishers, Inc., Oakland Ca.

Chapter 2

Baker, E.R. (1985) "Body weight and the initiation of puberty," *Clin Obstet Gynecol*, September, 28(3), 573–9. doi: 10.1097/00003081-198528030-00013. PMID: 4053451.

Dementia prevention, intervention, and care: 2024 report of the Lancet standing Commission Livingston, Gill et al. The Lancet, Volume 404, Issue 10452, 572–628

Harrison, Christy (2023) *The Wellness Trap: Break Free from Diet Culture, Disinformation, and Dubious Diagnoses, and Find Your True Well-Being*, Little, Brown, Spark.

Larocca, Amy. (2022, December 20). Welcome to the Menopause Gold Rush. *New York Times*, https://www.nytimes.com/2022/12/20/style/menopause-womens-health-goop.html

Chapter 3

Aubrey Gordon and Michael Hobbes (Producers). (2010, October 20). The President's Physical Fitness Test [Audio podcast]. Retrieved from https://maintenancephase.buzzsprout.com/1411126/episodes/5960191-the-president-s-physical-fitness-test

Cataldo, I., De Luca, I., Giorgetti, V., Cicconcelli, D., Bersani, F.S., Imperatori, C., Abdi, S., Negri, A., Esposito, G., & Corazza, O. (2021) "Fitspiration on social media: Body-image and other psychopathological risks among young adults: A narrative review," *Emerging Trends in Drugs, Addictions, and Health*, 1, 100010, ISSN 2667-1182, doi: 10.1016/j.etdah.2021.100010.

Crouse, L. (2022) "I ditched my smart watch, and I don't regret it," *New York Times*, January 28, https://www.nytimes.com/2022/01/28/opinion/smartwatch-health-body.html

Curtis, R.G., Prichard, I., Gosse, G. et al. (2023) "Hashtag fitspiration: Credibility screening and content analysis of Instagram fitness accounts," *BMC Public Health*, 23, 421. doi: 10.1186/s12889-023-15232-7

Friedman, D. (2023) "Most fitness influencers are doing more harm than good," *New York Times*, May 10, https://www.nytimes.com/2023/05/10/well/move/fitness-influencers.html

Janin, A. (2023) "What if the most powerful way to live longer is just exercise?" *Wall Street Journal*, June 12, https://www.wsj.com/health/fight-aging-science-research-146aa2cd

Jerónimo, F. & Carraça, E.V. (2022) "Effects of fitspiration content on body image: A systematic review," *Eat Weight Disord.*, December, 27(8), 3017–35. doi: 10.1007/s40519-022-01505-4. Epub 2022 Nov 18. PMID: 36401082; PMCID: PMC9676749.

Kendall, K.L, & Fairman, C.M. (2014) "Women and exercise in aging," *Journal of Sport and Health Science*, 3(3), 170–8, ISSN 2095-2546.

Lembke, Anna. (2023) *Dopamine Nation: Finding Balance in the Age of Indulgence*, Dutton.

Piran, N. (2019) *Handbook of Positive Body Image and Embodiment: Constructs, Protective Factors, and Interventions*, Oxford University Press.

Piran, N. & Neumark-Sztainer, D. (2020) "Yoga and the experience of embodiment: A discussion of possible links," *Eating Disorders: The Journal of Treatment & Prevention*, 28(4), 330–8.

Prichard, I., Kavanagh, E., Mulgrew, K.E., Lim, M.S.C., & Tiggemann, M. (2020) "The effect of Instagram #fitspiration images on young women's mood, body image, and exercise behaviour," *Body Image*, 33, 1–6. ISSN 1740-1445.

Wu, Y., Harford, J., Petersen, J., & Prichard, I. (2022) "'Eat clean, train mean, get lean': Body image and health behaviours of women who engage with fitspiration and clean eating imagery on Instagram," *Body Image*, 42, 25–31. doi: 10.1016/j.bodyim.2022.05.003. ISSN 1740-1445.

Chapter 4

Crawford, R. (1980). HEALTHISM AND THE MEDICALIZATION OF EVERYDAY LIFE. *International Journal of Health Services, 10*(3), 365–388. http://www.jstor.org/stable/45130677

McCleary-Gaddy, A.T., Miller, C.T., Grover, K.W., Hodge, J.J., & Major, B. (2019) "Weight stigma and hypothalamic-pituitary-adrenocortical axis reactivity in individuals who are overweight," *Ann Behav Med*, March 20, 53(4), 392–98. doi: 10.1093/abm/kay042. PMID: 29917036; PMCID: PMC6426042.

McMillan Cottom, T. (2019) *Thick: And Other Essays*, New Press.

Phelan, S.M., Burgess, D.J., Yeazel, M.W., Hellerstedt, W.L., Griffin, J.M., & van Ryn, M. (2015) "Impact of weight bias and stigma on quality of care and outcomes for patients with obesity," *Obes Rev*, April, 16(4), 319–26. doi: 10.1111/obr.12266. Epub 2015 Mar 5. PMID: 25752756; PMCID: PMC4381543.

Puhl, R.M. & Brownell, K.D. (2006) "Confronting and coping with weight stigma: An investigation of overweight and obese adults," *Obesity*, 14, 1802–15. doi: 10.1038/oby.2006.208

Samuels, K.L., Maine, M.M., & Tantillo, M. (2019) "Disordered eating: Eating disorders, and body image in midlife and older women," *Curr Psychiatry Rep.*, 21(8),70. doi: 10.1007/s11920-019-1057-5. PMID: 31264039.

Strings, Sabrina (2019). *Fearing the Black Body: The Racial Origins of Fat Phobia*. New York University Press.

Wolf, N. (2002) *The Beauty Myth*, Harper Perennial.

Wu, Y.-K. & Berry, D.C. (2018) "Impact of weight stigma on physiological and psychological health outcomes for overweight and obese adults: A systematic review," *J Adv Nurs.*, 74, 1030–42.

The Way Down: God, Greed, and the Cult of Gwen Shamblin, HBO, 2022.

Chapter 5

Ellyn Satter Institute, https://www.ellynsatterinstitute.org/

Kenney, W.L. & Chiu, P. (2001) "Influence of age on thirst and fluid intake," *Medicine & Science in Sports & Exercise*, September, 33(9), 1524–1532.

Martin, B. (2021) *The Art of Giving and Receiving: The Wheel of Consent*, Luminare Press.

Neff, K. (2003) "Self-compassion: An alternative conceptualization of a healthy attitude toward oneself," *Self and Identity*, 2(2), 85–101.

Schwartz, R. (2021) *No Bad Parts: Healing Trauma and Restoring Wholeness with the Internal Family Systems Model*, Vermillion.

They Starved So That Others Be Better Fed: Remembering Ancel Keys and the Minnesota Experiment Kalm, Leah M. et al. The Journal of Nutrition, Volume 135, Issue 6, 1347–1352

Tribole, E. & Resch, E. (2020) *Intuitive Eating: A Revolutionary Anti-Diet Approach*, St. Martin's Essentials.

Waheed, Nayyirah (2013) *Salt*. Self-published.

Chapter 6

Armitage, H (2019, 5 Questions: Gardner on the intersection of meat, protein and the environment [Blog post]. Retrieved from https://med.stanford.edu/news/all-news/2019/02/5-questions-gardner-on-meat-protein-and-environment.html

Davis, S. (2024) "Top nutrition and fitness trends in 2024, according to experts," *Forbes*, February 19.

Ding, H., Reiss, A.B., Pinkhasov, A., & Kasselman, L.J. (2022) "Plants, plants, and more plants: Plant-derived nutrients and their protective roles in cognitive function, Alzheimer's disease, and other dementias," *Medicina* (Kaunas), July 30, 58(8), 1025. doi: 10.3390/medicina58081025. PMID: 36013492; PMCID: PMC9414574. https://pubmed.ncbi.nlm.nih.gov/36013492/

Dominguez, L.J., Veronese, N., & Barbagallo, M. (2024) "Magnesium and the hallmarks of aging," *Nutrients*, February 9, 16(4), 496. doi:

10.3390/nu16040496. PMID: 38398820; PMCID: PMC10892939. https://pubmed.ncbi.nlm.nih.gov/38398820/

Ellyn Satter Institute. The Satter Division of Responsibility in Feeding https://www.ellynsatterinstitute.org/how-to-feed/the-division-of-responsibility-in-feeding/

La Berge, A.F. (2008) "How the ideology of low fat conquered America," *Journal of the History of Medicine and Allied Sciences*, April, 63(2), 139–77. doi: 10.1093/jhmas/jrn001

Livingston, G. et al. (2024) "Dementia prevention, intervention, and care: 2024 report of the Lancet Standing Commission," *The Lancet*, 404(10452), 572–628. https://www.thelancet.com/journals/lancet/article/PIIS0140-6736(24)01296-0/

Ritter S. Monitoring and Maintenance of Brain Glucose Supply: Importance of Hindbrain Catecholamine Neurons in This Multifaceted Task. In: Harris RBS, editor. Appetite and Food Intake: Central Control. 2nd edition. Boca Raton (FL): CRC Press/Taylor & Francis; 2017. Chapter 9.

Chapter 7

Brown, A.M. (2019) *Pleasure Activism: The Politics of Feeling Good*, AK Press.

CDC (MMWR) (2022) "QuickStats: Age-adjusted percentage* of adults aged ≥18 years who met the 2018 Federal Physical Activity Guidelines for both muscle-strengthening and aerobic physical activity,† by urbanization level§—National Health Interview Survey, United States, 2020," *Weekly*, July 8, 71(27), 887. https://www.cdc.gov/mmwr/volumes/71/wr/mm7127a6.htm

Gupta, S. (2021) *Keep Sharp: Build a Better Brain at Any Age*. Simon & Schuster.

Langhammer, B., Bergland, A., & Rydwik, E. (2018) "The importance of physical activity exercise among older people," *Biomed Res Int*, December 5, 7856823. doi: 10.1155/2018/7856823. PMID: 30627571; PMCID: PMC6304477. https://pubmed.ncbi.nlm.nih.gov/30627571/

Lichtenstein, M.B., Hinze, C.J., Emborg, B., Thomsen, F., & Hemmingsen, S.D. (2017) "Compulsive exercise: Links, risks and challenges faced," *Psychol Res Behav Manag*. March 30, 10, 85–95. doi: 10.2147/PRBM.S113093. PMID: 28435339; PMCID: PMC5386595. https://pubmed.ncbi.nlm.nih.gov/28435339/

Maine, M., Ph.D. & Kelly, J. (2016) *Pursuing Perfection: Eating Disorders, Body Myths, and Women at Midlife and Beyond*, Routledge.

Palus, S. (2023) "The last exercise column you ever need to read," *Slate*, December 22.

Palus, Shannon. (2023, December 22). The Last Exercise Column You Ever Need to Read. *Slate*. Retrieved from https://slate.com/technology/2023/12/last-exercise-column-you-ever-need.html

Schnohr, P., O'Keefe, J., Marott, J. et al. (2015) "Dose of jogging and long-term mortality: The Copenhagen City Heart Study," *JACC*, February, 65(5), 411–19.

Chapter 8

Dana, D. (2018) *The Polyvagal Theory in Therapy: Engaging the Rhythm of Regulation* (Norton Series on Interpersonal Neurobiology), WW Norton & Co.

Hersey, Tricia (2024) *Rest Is Resistance: Free yourself from grind culture and reclaim your life*, Aster.

Hirshkowitz, M., Whiton, K., Albert, S.M., Alessi, C., Bruni, O., DonCarlos, L., Hazen, N., Herman, J., Katz, E.S., Kheirandish-Gozal, L., Neubauer, D.N., O'Donnell, A.E., Ohayon, M., Peever, J., Rawding, R., Sachdeva, R.C., Setters, B., Vitiello, M.V., Ware, J.C., & Adams Hillard, P.J. (2015) "National Sleep Foundation's sleep time duration recommendations: Methodology and results summary," *Sleep Health*, March, 1(1), 40–3. doi: 10.1016/j.sleh.2014.12.010. Epub 2015 Jan 8. PMID: 29073412. https://pubmed.ncbi.nlm.nih.gov/29073412/

Ohayon, M., Wickwire, E.M., Hirshkowitz, M., Albert, S.M., Avidan, A., Daly, F.J., Dauvilliers, Y., Ferri, R., Fung, C., Gozal, D., Hazen, N., Krystal, A., Lichstein, K., Mallampalli, M., Plazzi, G., Rawding, R., Scheer, F.A., Somers, V., & Vitiello, M.V. (2017) "National Sleep Foundation's sleep quality recommendations: First report," *Sleep Health*, February, 3(1), 6–19. doi: 10.1016/j.sleh.2016.11.006. Epub 2016 Dec 23. PMID: 28346153.

Raheem, Octavia (2024) *Rest Is Sacred: Reclaiming Our Brilliance through the Practice of Stillness.* Shambhala.

Rees, A., Wiggins, M.W., Helton, W.S., Loveday, T., & O'Hare, D. (2017) "The impact of breaks on sustained attention in a simulated, semi-automated train control task," *Appl. Cognit. Psychol.*, 31, 351–9. doi: 10.1002/acp.3334.

See Pause Playlist on Deb Benfield's Spotify https://open.spotify.com/user/dlbenfield?si=57288312eb154ee6

Siegel, Dan. (2020) *The Developing Mind: How Relationships and the Brain Interact to Shape Who We Are*, The Guilford Press.

Van der Kolk, Bessel (2015) *The Body Keep the Score: Brain, Mind, and Body in the Healing of Trauma*, Penguin.

Chapter 9

DePaulo, Bella (2023) *Single at Heart: The Power, Freedom, and Heart-Filling Joy of Single Life*, Apollo Publishers.

Doll, G. (2023) "I saw it in the movies: Accurate representations of older adult sexuality in films," *Generations Journal*, Winter 2022–23. https://generations.asaging.org/accurate-film-representations-elder-sexuality

Gelles-Watnick, R. (2023) "For Valentine's Day, 5 facts about single Americans," Pew Research Center, February 8. https://www.pewresearch.org/short-reads/2023/02/08/for-valentines-day-5-facts-about-single-americans/ft_2023-02-08_facts-single-americans_01-png/

Kwee, Janelle & McBride, Hillary Ed. (2018), *Embodiment and Eating Disorders: Theory, Research, Prevention and Treatment*, Routledge.

McBride, Hillary (2021) *The Wisdom of Your Body: Finding Healing, Wholeness, and Connection through Embodied Living*, Brazos.

Nagoski, E. (2025) *Come Together: The Science (and Art) of Creating Lasting Sexual Connections*, Ballentine Books.

Nagoski, E. (2021) *Come As You Are: The Surprising New Science That Will Transform Your Sex Life*, Simon & Schuster.

O'Donohue, J. (2022) "The inner landscape of beauty," *On Being* podcast with Krista Tippett, January 10. https://onbeing.org/programs/john-odonohue-the-inner-landscape-of-beauty/

Orth, U., Erol, R.Y., & Luciano, E.C. (2018) "Development of self-esteem from age 4 to 94 years: A meta-analysis of longitudinal studies," *Psychological Bulletin*, 144(10), 1045–80. https://doi.org/10.1037/bul0000161

Park, Y., Page-Gould, E., & MacDonald, G. (2022) "Satisfying singlehood as a function of age and cohort: Satisfaction with being single increases with age after midlife," *Psychol Aging,* August, 37(5), 626–36. doi: 10.1037/pag0000695. Epub 2022 Jun 16. PMID: 35708941. https://pubmed.ncbi.nlm.nih.gov/35708941/

Pujols, Y., Seal, B.N., & Meston, C.M. (2010) "The association between sexual satisfaction and body image in women," *J Sex Med.*, February, 7(2 Pt 2), 905–16. doi: 10.1111/j.1743-6109.2009.01604.x. Epub 2009 Nov 24. Erratum in: J Sex Med. 2010 Jun;7(6):2295. PMID: 19968771; PMCID: PMC2874628. https://pmc.ncbi.nlm.nih.gov/articles/PMC2874628/

Schaller, S.L., Kvalem, I.L., & Træen, B. (2023) "Constructions of sexual identities in the ageing body: A qualitative exploration of older Norwegian adults: Negotiation of body image and sexual satisfaction," *Sexuality & Culture*, 27, 1369–1402. doi: 10.1007/s12119-023-10067-1

Chapter 10

Applewhite, A. (2020) *This Chair Rocks: A Manifesto Against Ageism*, Celadon Books.

Becker, C.B., Middlemass, K., Taylor, B., Johnson, C., & Gomez, F. (2017) "Food insecurity and eating disorder pathology," *Int J Eat Disord.*, September, 50(9), 1031–40. doi: 10.1002/eat.22735. Epub 2017 Jun 18. PMID: 28626944. https://pubmed.ncbi.nlm.nih.gov/28626944/

Black MM, Aboud FE. Responsive feeding is embedded in a theoretical framework of responsive parenting. J Nutr. 2011 Mar;141(3):490–4. doi: 10.3945/jn.110.129973. Epub 2011 Jan 26. PMID: 21270366; PMCID: PMC3040905.

Brun, I., Russell-Mayhew, S., & Mudry, T. (2020) "Last word: Ending the intergenerational transmission of body dissatisfaction and disordered eating: A call to investigate the mother–daughter relationship," *Eating Disorders*, 29(6), 591–8. doi: 10.1080/10640266.2020.1712635 de Jorge, M.C., Rukh, G., Williams, M.J., Gaudio, S., Brooks, S., & Helgi B. Schiöth, (2022) "Genetics of anorexia nervosa: An overview of genome-wide association studies and emerging biological links," *Journal of Genetics and Genomics*, 49(1), 1–12, ISSN 1673–8527. https://www.sciencedirect.com/science/article/abs/pii/S1673852721003209?via%3Dihub

Deek, M.R., Prichard, I., & Kemps, E. (2023) "The mother–daughter–sister triad: The role of female family members in predicting body image and eating behaviour in young women," *Body Image*, 46, 336–46. doi: 10.1016/j.bodyim.2023.07.001. ISSN 1740-1445,

Dias, B. & Ressler, K. (2014) "Parental olfactory experience influences behavior and neural structure in subsequent generations," *Nat Neurosci.*, 17, 89–96. doi: 10.1038/nn.3594

ESI (n.d.) "Raise a child who is a joy to feed," Ellyn Satter Institute: Division of Responsibility. https://www.ellynsatterinstitute.org/how-to-feed/the-division-of-responsibility-in-feeding

Hübel, C., Marzi, S.J., Breen, G., & Bulik, C.M. (2019) "Epigenetics in eating disorders: A systematic review," *Mol Psychiatry*, June, 24(6), 901–15. doi: 10.1038/s41380-018-0254-7. Epub 2018 Oct 23. PMID: 30353170; PMCID: PMC6544542. https://pubmed.ncbi.nlm.nih.gov/30353170/

Lerner, H. (2017) *Why Won't You Apologize? Healing Big Betrayals and Everyday Hurts*, Gallery Books.

Loth, K.A., Uy, M.J.A., Winkler, M.R., Neumark-Sztainer, D., Fisher, J.O., & Berge, J.M. (2019) "The intergenerational transmission of family meal practices: A mixed-methods study of parents of young children," *Public Health Nutr.*, May, 22(7), 1269–80. doi: 10.1017/S1368980018003920. Epub 2019 Feb 8. PMID: 30732660; PMCID: PMC6715132. https://pubmed.ncbi.nlm.nih.gov/30732660/

Rosebloom, T.J., Painter, R.C., van Abeelen, A.F., Veenendaal, M.V., & de Rooij, S.R. (2011) "Hungry in the womb: What are the consequences? Lessons from the Dutch famine," *Maturitas*, October, 70(2), 141–5. doi: 10.1016/j.maturitas.2011.06.017. Epub 2011 Jul 28. PMID: 21802226. https://pubmed.ncbi.nlm.nih.gov/21802226/

Sole-Smith, Virginia (2023) *Fat Talk: Parenting in the Age of Diet Culture*, Henry Holt and Co.

Schwartz, R. (n.d.) "Evolution of the Internal Family Systems Model," IFS Institute. https://ifs-institute.com/resources/articles/evolution-internal-family-systems-model-dr-richard-schwartz-ph-d

Schwartz, R. (2021) *No Bad Parts*, Vermilion.

Thaler, L. & Steiger, H. (2017) "Eating disorders and epigenetics," *Adv Exp Med Biol.*, 978, 93–103. doi: 10.1007/978-3-319-53889-1_5. PMID: 28523542. https://pubmed.ncbi.nlm.nih.gov/28523542/

Resources

I've read and studied hundreds of books, articles, and podcasts and tried my best to vet and share resources free of ageism, anti-aging, and anti-fat bias. Sadly, few met my standards, so I included resources I found *mostly* helpful. I am sorry if I missed something in these resources, and I hope this list will continue to grow!

Books on ageism/aging/death

Applewhite, Ashton, *This Chair Rocks: A Manifesto Against Ageism*, Celdaon Books, 2019.

Arthur, Alua, *Briefly Perfectly Human: Making an Authentic Life by Getting Real About the End*, Mariner Books, 2024.

Gendron, Tracey, Ph.D., *Ageism Unmasked: Exploring Age Bias and How to End It*, Steerforth, 2022.

Levy, Becca, Ph.D., *Breaking the Age Code: How Your Beliefs About Aging Determine How Long and Well You Live*, William Morrow, 2022.

Mannix, Kathryn, *With the End in Mind: Dying, Death, and Wisdom in an Age of Denial*, Little, Brown Spark, 2018.

Moon, Susan, *Alive Until You're Dead: Notes on the Home Stretch*, Shambhala, 2022.

Pipher, Mary, *Women Rowing North: Navigating Life's Currents and Flourishing as We Age*, Bloomsbury, 2019.

Steinke, Darcey, *Flash Count Diary: Menopause and the Vindication of Natural Life*, Sarah Crichton Books, 2019.

Walrond, Karen, *Radiant Rebellion: Reclaim Aging, Practice Joy, and Raise a Little Hell*, Broadleaf Books, 2023.

Books on non-diet/midlife eating disorders/ body liberation

Brown, Adrienne Maree (ed.), *Pleasure Activism: The Politics of Feeling Good*, AK Press, 2019.

Bulik, Cynthia, Ph.D., *Midlife Eating Disorders: Your Journey to Recovery*, Walker and Company, 2013.

Dillon, Julie Duffy, *Find Your Food Voice: Defy Diet Culture, Declare Body Liberation, and Reclaim Your Peace*, Sheldon Press, 2025.

Harrison, Christy, *Anti-Diet: Reclaim Your Time, Money, Well-Being, and Happiness Through Intuitive Eating* Little, Brown Spark, 2019.

—*The Wellness Trap: Break Free from Diet Culture, Disinformation, and Dubious Diagnoses, and Find Your True Well-Being*, Little, Brown Spark, 2023.

Hemphill, Prentis, *What It Takes to Heal: How Transforming Ourselves Can Change the World*, Random House, 2024.

King, Chrissy, *The Body Liberation Project: How Understanding Racism and Diet Culture Helps Cultivate Joy and Build Collective Freedom*, Tiny Reparations Books, 2023.

Kinsey, Dalia, *Decolonizing Wellness: A QTBIPOC-Centered Guide to Escape the Diet Trap, Heal Your Self-Image, and Achieve Body Liberation*, BenBella Books, 2022.

Maine, Margo, Ph.D. and Joe Kelly, *Pursuing Perfection: Eating Disorders, Body Myths, and Women at Midlife and Beyond*, Routledge, 2016.

Manne, Kate Ph.D., *Unshrinking: How to Face Fat Phobia*, Crown, 2024.

McCullough, Alisha, *Reclaiming the Black Body: Nourishing the Home Within*, The Dial Press, 2025.

Schauster, Heidi, *Nourish: How to Heal Your Relationship with Food, Body, and Self*, Self-Published, 2018.

Spence, Shana, *Live Nourished: Make Peace with Food, Banish Body Shame, and Reclaim Joy*, S&S/Simon Element, 2024.

Spinks, Sawanda, *Weightless Wisdom: How to Break Free From Diet Culture and Embrace Your NOW Body*, Self-Published, 2024.

Sturdevant, Dana and Kinavey, Hilary, *Reclaiming Body Trust: A Path to Healing and Liberation*, TarcherPerigee, 2022.

Tribole, Evelyn and Resch, Elyse, *Intuitive Eating: A Revolutionary Anti-Diet Approach*, St. Martin's Essentials, 2020.

Books on healing intergenerational diet culture

Brooks, Sumner and Severson, Amee, *How to Raise an Intuitive Eater: Raising the Next Generation with Food and Body Confidence*, St. Martin's Essentials, 2022.

Schauster, Heidi, *Nurture: How to Raise Kids Who Love Food, Their Bodies, and Themselves*, Self-Published, 2024.

Sole-Smith, Virginia, *Fat Talk: Parenting in the Age of Diet Culture*, Henry Holt and Co., 2023.

Books on body image/relationship

Kite, Lexie and Kite, Lindsay, *More Than a Body: Your Body Is an Instrument, Not an Ornament*, Harvest, 2020.

Markey, Charlotte, Ph.D., *Adultish: The Body Image Book for Life*, Cambridge University Press, 2024.

Piran, Niva, *Journeys of Embodiment at the Intersection of Body and Culture: The Developmental Theory of Embodiment*, Academic Press, 2017.

Taylor, Sonya Renee, *The Body Is Not an Apology: The Power of Radical Self-Love*, Berett-Koehler Publishers, 2021.

Tylka, Tracy L. and Piran, Niva (eds.) *Handbook of Positive Body Image and Embodiment: Constructs, Protective Factors, and Interventions*, Oxford University Press, 2019.

Books on embodiment, sexuality, and movement

Daly, Niamh, *Yoga for Menopause and Beyond: Guiding Teachers and Students Through Change*, Human Kinetics, 2024.

Guest-Jelley, Anna, *Curvy Yoga: Love Yourself & Your Body a Little More Each Day*, Union Square & Co., 2017.

Heyman, Jivana, *Accessible Yoga Poses and Practices for Every Body*, Shambhala, 2019.

McBride, Hillary L., Ph.D., *Practices for Embodied Living: Experiencing the Wisdom of Your Body*, Brazos, 2024.

Ngoski, Emily, *Come Together: The Science (and Art) of Creating Lasting Sexual Connections*, Ballentine Books, 2025.

Ngoski, Emily, *Come As You Are: The Surprising New Science That Will Transform Your Sex Life*, Simon & Schuster, 2021.

Reardon, Sara, Ph.D., *Floored: A Woman's Guide to Pelvic Floor Health at Every Age and Stage*, Park Row, 2025.

Stanley, Jessamyn, *Every Body Yoga: Let Go of Fear, Get on Your Mat, Love Your Body*, Workman Publishing Company, 2017.

Books on body biases

Brown, Harriet, *Body of Truth: How Science, History, and Culture Drive Our Obsession with Weight – and What We Can Do About It*, Balance, 2015.

Gordon, Aubrey, *"You Just Need to Lose Weight": and 19 Other Myths About Fat People*, Beacon Press, 2023.

—*What We Don't Talk About When We Talk About Fat*, Beacon, 2020.

Harrison, Da'Shaun, L. *Belly of the Beast: The Politics of Anti-Fatness as Anti-Blackness*, North Atlantic Books, 2021.

McMillan Cottom, Tressie, Ph.D., *Thick: And Other Essays*, The New Press, 2019.

Nordell, Jessica, *The End of Bias: A Beginning: The Science and Practice of Overcoming Unconscious Bias*, Metropolitan Books, 2021.

Piepzna-Samarasinha, Leah Lakshmi, *Care Work: Dreaming Disability Justice*, Arsenal Pulp Press, 2018.

Strings, Sabrina, Ph.D., *Fearing the Black Body: The Origins of Fat Phobia*, NYU Press, 2019.

Wilson, Jessica, *It's Always Been Ours: Rewriting the Story of Black Women's Bodies*, Balance, 2023.

Wong, Alice, *Disability Visibility: First-Person Stories from the Twenty-First Century*, Vintage, 2020.

Park Y, Page-Gould E, MacDonald G. Satisfying singlehood as a function of age and cohort: Satisfaction with being single increases with age after midlife. Psychol Aging. 2022 Aug;37(5):626–636. doi: 10.1037/pag0000695. Epub 2022 Jun 16. PMID: 35708941.

Orth, U., Erol, R. Y., & Luciano, E. C. (2018). Development of self-esteem from age 4 to 94 years: A meta-analysis of longitudinal studies. Psychological Bulletin, 144(10), 1045–1080.

Common Sense Media (2020, June 04) At what age does media begin affecting my child's body image. https://www.commonsensemedia.org/press-releases/new-report-by-common-sense-media-reveals-kids-body-image-develops-as-early-as-five-and-media-and-parents

Podcasts

Ageism Is Never in Style with Jacynth Bassett

Body Liberation for All with Dalia Kinsey

Burnt Toast with Virginia Sole-Smith

Eat the Rules with Summer Innanen

Food Psych with Christy Harrison

Maintenance Phase with Audrey Gordon and Michael Hobbes

Rethinking Wellness with Christy Harrison

Making It Awkward with Jessica Wilson

Wiser Than Me with Julia Louis-Dreyfus

Find Your Food Voice with Julie Duffy Dillon

The Body Trust Podcast with Dana Sturtevant, Hilary Kinavey, and Sirius Bonner

The Midlife Feast with Jenn Salib Huber

The Full Plate Podcast with Abbie Attwood

Interviews with the author: debrabenfield.com/media

Interviews with Ragen Chastain

Interviews with Tracey Gendron, Ashton Applewhite, and Becca Levy

Other resources

Old School: A Hub for Age Equity and Ageism Awareness: old-school.info

Association for Size Diversity and Health (ASDAH): asdah.org

Dances with Fat: danceswithfat.org

Unapologetic Aging: debbenfield.substack.com

David Wilson on Instagram: @oldscoolmoves

Parenting without diet culture: oonahanson.substack.com

Foot health: gaithappens.com

Project Implicit: https://implicit.harvard.edu/implicit/takeatest.html

Additional practices/rituals/journaling prompts can be found at: debrabenfield.com/practices

Acknowledgments

First, I would like to acknowledge that I created this work on the land of the Catawba, Cheraw, Keuyauwee, Tutelo, and Occaneechi tribes in what is now Winston-Salem, North Carolina.

My learning has come primarily from my clients, who sat across from me in individual sessions, yoga classes, workshops, groups, and memberships and shared their pain, sorrows, and joys about their bodies. I am honored and deeply grateful for the trust you placed in me and yourselves and the ways you showed up for yourselves and our work together. This book would not exist without you.

I have learned so much from the work of activists and teachers in the anti-ageism and anti-fat bias fields and all realms of body liberation, including Ashton Applewhite, Becca Levy, Sonya Renee Taylor, Jacynth Bassett, Tigress Osborn, Kate Manne, Alisha McCullough, Deb Burgard, Sharon Maxwell, Rachel Millner, Marilyn Wann, Da'Shaun Harrison, Kiese Laymon, Harriett Brown, Chevese Turner, Paul Campos, Dana Sturdevant, Hilary Kinavy, Hillary McBride, Sabrina Strings, Christy Harrison, Aubrey Gordon, Ragen Chastain, Elyse Resch, Evelyn Tribole, Jessica Wilson, and Chrissy King. I'm profoundly grateful for my conversations with Meg Bradbury, Karen Samuels, David Wilson, Tracey Gendron, Karen Walrond, Oona Hanson, Margo Maine, Virginia Sole-Smith, Niamh Daly, Anna Fleig, Cheyenne Carter, and Sawanda Spinks.

I cannot say enough how much I appreciate the support of my small but mighty Diet Disruptors writing group, Julie Duffy Dillon and Heidi Schauster. Our shared vision and your consistent presence and messages of encouragement meant the world to me and sometimes helped me get my butt back in my chair. Thank you to everyone who contributed to and supported my work on this book, especially Rachel Landes and everyone at Sheldon Press.

I could not have written this book without the support of the big-hearted and whip-smart Registered Dietitians in my group practice: Jane Anderson Weiss, MPH, RDN, LDN; Andrea Tsavahidis Lawrence, MS, RDN, LDN; and Katie Wolf, MPH, RDN, LDN. Thank you for caring for our clients and colleagues and offering consultation to our community. I appreciate your steadfast support and all the ways you stepped up so I could continue writing. Feeling confident that our clients are in such good hands is priceless.

I appreciate the hours of listening to my first-time author trials and lessons on our many walks and talks this year with dear friends Betsy Reiner, Seth Kratwurst, Camille Izlar, and Mary Jane Elliott. I also owe much gratitude to my sister Denise Yost and aunt Janice Wall, who cared for my mother so I could devote my time and energy to writing. Those who care make the world go round.

Creating our Unapologetically Aging Community was my first spark, vision, and end goal. Our community continues to be where all these ideas take root in the hearts and lives of humans traveling and thriving together in midlife and beyond. I adore the way we valiantly resist the pressures to control and contain ourselves. A big thank you to my newsletter readers, who participated in conversations and responded to my questions throughout this process.

My boundless love and thanks to my sons and daughter-in-law. You have been my life's greatest teachers and enlarged my heart's capacity like no other. Thank you for your creative and spacious spirits, inspiring me to bring my own. And above all, I wrote this book for my grandchildren, Chloe and Bridget. I hope you grow up knowing your body is your partner, your home, and not the source of your worthiness.

Index

Join the Sheldon Press community today, sign up for our newsletter!

- Select a **FREE eBook** or extract to read upon joining

- Keep up with our latest publishing and exciting author news

- Be the first to hear about book prize draws, free extracts, and upcoming author events

Simply scan the QR code below or head to www.sheldonpress.co.uk/newsletter to sign up.

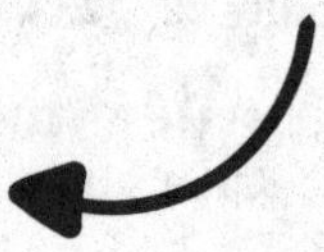